Contents

Meet the contributors

Sarah Adams

Sarah is a practice nurse working in Nottinghamshire. She has extensive experience in diabetes, asthma and all aspects of practice nursing. Her main interests include endocrinology and specialist practice.

Mick Ashman

Mick is a nursing lecturer at the University of Sheffield. He teaches on critical care and has a particular interest in management issues within healthcare and nursing.

Chris Bassett

Chris is a lecturer in acute and critical care at the University of Sheffield. He has an enduring interest in the issues surrounding clinical supervision. He writes widely for the British and international press and has lectured in Europe, North America and Australia. He has edited a major new text on high dependency care and is in the process of editing a text for EMAP Healthcare on research utilisation. He is also preparing an exciting new text on practice development.

Nicola Clibbens

Nicola has worked as a RMN in acute inpatient psychiatric care since 1989. She has studied part time throughout her career. She recently completed an MA in Education and registered as a nurse teacher. She currently has a joint appointment between the University of Sheffield and Community Health Care Services, North Derbyshire NHS Trust as a practice development adviser. In the trust role Nicola is responsible for promoting evidence-based practice and encouraging innovation in clinical practice within mental health services. She has taken a lead in the implementation of clinical supervision in the trust and continues to develop clinical supervision in mental health across both the trust and the university.

Deborah Glover

Deborah qualified in 1983 at University College Hospital, London. Clinical areas she has worked in include care of the elderly, oncology, ITU and HIV. Over the past few years she has been involved in practice and professional development roles and has brought her clinical and development experiences to her post as clinical editor for Nursing Times. Deborahís main passion is the development of practice that retains the values and principles of nursing. She also has a more than passing interest in accountability and legal issues in nursing and is the author of an NT Clinical Monograph on the subject, available on 01483 303017.

Mac Macintosh

Mac is a lecturer in the Department of Acute and Critical Care Nursing at the University of Sheffield. Since 1992 he has been involved in the education and development of nurses at all levels in the field of coronary care and cardiac nursing. He teaches management and leadership to practising nurses undertaking post-registration education and has a particular interest in the use of outdoor activities in leadership development. He has recently registered to study for a PhD for which he will be exploring interventions to reduce patient delay in reporting symptoms of heart attack.

Robert McSherry

Since qualifying in 1988, Robert has worked in acute care of the elderly, rehabilitation and stroke rehabilitation wards, gaining invaluable theoretical, clinical, managerial and organisational experience within nursing. He is a senior lecturer in adult nursing in the practice and professional development team at the University of Teeside, Middlesborough. His long-term aim is to develop and strengthen practice and professional development within the school of health and in NHS trusts in Teeside. For five years he was practice development adviser, medical specialities directorate at Chesterfield Royal Hospital NHS Trust, where he facilitated and supported the introduction of research. His main interest is research utilisation at a clinical level where nurses, midwives, nurse specialists and other professionals are equipped with the essential skills and knowledge to aid this process.

1 Introduction and background

Chris Bassett

Clinical supervision is an idea that has come of age. When one considers the pressures placed on nurses in all areas of practice today, it is little wonder that we are in the midst of a serious situation in nursing with falling recruitment and a marked increase in nurses leaving the service (Agnew, 1998). For many years I have thought that the internal culture of not only nursing but also healthcare in general was just not caring enough towards those of us who work within it. We are all here to provide the best care for our patients. The healthcare system in the United Kingdom is, without doubt, providing a very good standard of care for the patients and clients experiencing ill health. This is not always necessarily the case relating to care given to the nursing staff working within the system. Levels of occupational stress are high and increasing. This situation, if ignored, may lead to an increase in stress-related illness and a worsening in the generally poor level of motivation and morale that exists. Increasingly, I hear from nurses that they do not enjoy their work as much as they did when they qualified. They seem to have lost their initial idealism. They have begun to feel that the stresses and pressures of nursing, that have perhaps always been present, are now just too much. As a consequence, many are looking for alternative employment outside the healthcare system (Lipley and Stokes, 1998). If one agrees with this analysis, then what is needed is a significant change to the culture within healthcare.

The good news is that a long-awaited shift in emphasis is occurring; there are distinct and important signs of optimism. Organisations are beginning to create internal systems of support for their staff; counselling services are present in many trusts. Trusts are beginning to learn that to get the best from staff, time for clinical supervision must be made. All staff must be helped and encouraged to develop personally and professionally. Nurses need time to improve their understanding of the changing context of health. Furthermore, they need time for personal reflection and education. Clinical supervision will help to enable the release of the great potential existing within our nurses. Clinical supervision for British nurses is a highly significant development that, if given time and encouragement by all parties, will help support the changes in culture that have already begun. In addition to helping to reduce the worst effects of stress and pressure, effective clinical supervision has another great potential benefit – it is a very potent educational tool. Nurses today are required by their code of conduct to develop their practice through development and education. The requirement for professional updating is made clear in the Post Registration Education and Practice Project (PREP) (UKCC, 1994). Clinical supervision has a great potential to tie together the PREP requirements of education and reflection that modern nursing practice requires to move forward. Clinical supervision asks nurses to explore practice and then reflect on the very basis of nursing care. This process can therefore provide valuable material for the personal professional profile that we are all required to keep as part of our re-registration commitment. Unfortunately, in many areas of practice there are still considerable constraints preventing widespread introduction of clinical supervision. This is acknowledged by the contributors to this book who are all committed to helping busy nurses, managers and healthcare professionals to get clinical supervision into practice.

There are a growing number of books and articles exploring the theoretical aspects of clinical supervision. In my experience, however, they tend to take an excessively theoretical approach. Surprisingly, very little literature actually considers the practicalities of introducing supervision into practice. This book is specifically designed to help the reader, whether nurse or ward manager, to implement clinical supervision in their area of practice.

To help the practitioner in implementing supervision the text will follow a logical approach. The authors (who are all experts in their field) will consider the subject in an open and accessible way. The benefits of supervision will be explored and differing models and approaches of supervision will then be examined and compared. Barriers to change will be identified and ways of overcoming these barriers will be considered. It is hoped that this will enable the practitioner to steer and manage the implementation of supervision to a successful conclusion. To underpin the content of the chapters, practice scenarios are used. This approach assists the reader in understanding the key issues and offers practical solutions to commonly experienced problems in the implementation of clinical supervision.

THE BACKGROUND TO CLINICAL SUPERVISION

For many years, there has been a pressing need for the creation of a system of internal dialogue between all practitioners of nursing. However, it is only in the comparatively recent past that a formalised system of clinical supervision has been proposed. For some time, formal clinical supervision has been integrated in disciplines other than nursing. Social work, for instance, has had supervision since the 1970s. Middleman and Rhodes (1985) state that social work supervision has nine functions: humanising, managing tension, catalysing, teaching, career socialising, evaluating, administrating, changing and advocating. I would argue that this list of aims for clinical supervision in social work is also a very appropriate list for nursing practice today.

Clinical supervision in nursing stems from several key documents, all outlining the need for a system of support.

KEY DOCUMENTS

Several important documents have been published outlining the ways that supervision would support and enhance nursing care. These include:

▶ Vision for the Future (Department of Health, 1993);

▶ Clothier Report;

▶ Delphi Study of Optimum Practice (Butterworth, 1994);

▶ Position Statement on Clinical Supervision (UKCC, 1995).

Statements from these documents include:

'Clinical supervision is necessary in clinical practice to enable practitioners to establish, maintain and promote standards and innovations in practice in the interests of patients and clients.' (UKCC, 1995)

'The exploration of the concept of clinical supervision of practitioners other than midwives should be further developed so that it is integral throughout the lifeline of practice, thus enabling practitioners to accept personal responsibility for and keep that care under constant review.' (Department of Health, 1993).

It is clear that clinical supervision has the potential to help us improve the ways that we work in the various clinical settings. It has a high level of support from both governmental and professional bodies who believe that clinical supervision, if implemented successfully, can help nurses care for their patients and clients more effectively.

The United Kingdom Central Council's position

In 1996 the United Kingdom Central Council (UKCC) issued a further position paper stating its views on clinical supervision. In this paper the UKCC placed clinical supervision in context. It stated that the kind of support that is part of clinical supervision has been available to some practitioners for years, but only on an ad hoc basis. Therefore, it felt that clinical supervision was needed to ensure that there was a comprehensive system in place that would benefit all practitioners. It considered that clinical supervision would have the potential to impact on and enhance vital practice issues such as:

- clinical risk management;
- enhancing staff morale;
- aiding recruitment;
- assisting in development of skills, knowledge and professional values;
- allowing practitioners to develop deeper understanding of what it is to be truly accountable for one's practice.

If combined, all of the above can enhance patient care through the systematic creation of a supportive and comprehensive system of clinical supervision for practitioners, wherever they practice.

WHAT IS CLINICAL SUPERVISION?

It is important to have an understanding of the meaning of clinical supervision. Many practitioners have commented on the term 'clinical supervision' in a negative way. Some believe that this phrase carries with it a certain claustrophobic feeling. It is as if someone is monitoring or watching your performance, measuring and recording what you do in your role. This, however, is not at all what clinical supervision is about.

Faugier and Butterworth (1993) offer us this definition of clinical supervision:

'An exchange between practising professionals to enable the development of professional knowledge and skills.'

The UKCC (1995) described clinical supervision as being 'a way to bring practitioners and skilled supervisors together to reflect on practice, with supervision aiming to identify solutions to problems, improve practice and increase understanding of professional issues.' It states that clinical supervision is not a managerial control system, and therefore nor is it:

▶ the exercise of overt managerial responsibility or managerial supervision;

▶ a system of formal individual performance review;

▶ hierarchical in nature.

The National Health Service Management Executive said this about clinical supervision:

'Clinical supervision is a term used to describe a formal process of professional support and learning which enables individual practitioners to develop knowledge and competence, assume responsibility for their own practice and enhance consumer protection and safety of care in complex clinical situations. It is central to the process of learning, to the expansion of the scope of practice and should be seen as a means of encouraging assessment, analytical and reflective skills.' (Department of Health, 1993)

It must be remembered that in order for clinical supervision to be effective and fully integrated into practice a committed management approach is essential.

PRINCIPLES OF CLINICAL SUPERVISION

From the above definitions of clinical supervision it is important to develop basic principles relating to its use and success.

▶ Supervision should become part and parcel of professional nursing practice.

▶ It should begin with basic professional education and continue as an integral part of professional development.

▶ It requires time, commitment and energy, and is not an incidental event.

▶ Organisational commitment is implicit. Supervision is protected in times of financial difficulty.

▶ Clinical supervision does not have one model but should be flexible.

▶ Practitioners must develop their own ways of supervising each other.

▶ It is locally led.

BARRIERS TO CLINICAL SUPERVISION

It would be quite wrong to approach the writing of this book from a position of having no practical experience or knowledge of the issues relating to the implementation of clinical supervision. Indeed the whole point of the book is to help practitioners implement supervision. In order to be successful in innovation it is essential that the difficulties relating to its implementation are made implicit. After spending several hundred hours training nurses in supervision, I believe the key issues relating to implementation for many nurses are the following:

'We don't have time to implement clinical supervision.'

The main concern raised in almost all training sessions is how the participants will find the time to implement clinical supervision. As previously mentioned, the workload in many practice areas has increased significantly. Staff levels are often lower than safe levels might dictate. PREP requirements (profiling and study) are also competing for any spare time.

'We already do clinical supervision.'

Many practitioners state that it already exists on an ad hoc basis for most staff anyway so 'in our unit/ward we do not actually need it'. Certainly, the last thing that the writers of this book would want would be the dismantling of existing professional links. However, nursing does need a comprehensive approach to supervision that allows time for all members of the team to have these discussions and benefits.

'I don't know how to be a supervisor or how to reflect on practice.'

There is a common belief that nurses are not prepared educationally to clinically supervise their colleagues. They are often not comfortable with concepts of support, counselling or reflective practice. This is possibly true, however I believe that nursing education and practice experience will give the practitioner something of a head start in communicating effectively with colleagues. It is, of course, essential that to make supervision successful both supervisors and supervised will need specific training to be efficient in their new roles. Reflection on practice is also a new concept for many but with some input and simple guidelines, reflective practice can be taught.

UNDERSTANDING REFLECTION

This aspect of nursing has become very important in recent years. There has been much written on the subject, indeed the literature abounds with articles on reflective practice. You are, of course, recommended to read widely around the subject of reflection. However, here are some simple guidelines relating to reflection.

Reflection, clinical supervision and you

Reflection on your practice during supervision will:

▶ allow you to consider the more hidden dimensions and issues relating to professional practice;

▶ help you challenge the issues relating to how we practice;

▶ help you ask searching questions of the individual;

▶ support you in deeper exploration of the self, increasing your awareness of personal strengths and weaknesses.

Issues surrounding reflection

Reflecting therefore might be defined as thinking purposefully about clinical practice to gain new insight, ideas and understanding. You need to understand that the benefits from structured reflection can be great, as it may shed light on alternate approaches to care (Haddock and Bassett, 1997). It may be that part of your clinical supervision session could form the basis of a reflective passage for your personal professional portfolio. Indeed I like to point out that it is here that we can save time, as our supervision sessions will provide a rich source of material for our profiles. You do not necessarily need to write very much to record reflective insights in your profile – short notes will often suffice, clearly summarising the key issues and possible ways forward. On the second point, you can gain confidence in reflecting by reading around the subject. Your skills will develop gradually over time, just as your nursing skills have developed. It should be remembered that there are no absolute rights or wrongs with reflecting on practice – just do what suits you. Very often you can crystallise the key issues of an event during supervision by writing them down. There is always some time that you can find to reflect on your supervision time and soon reflection will become a valuable part of your professional life.

In addition to the above issues preventing clinical supervision, there may be other less obvious reasons for nurses resisting supervision. These were identified by Wilkin et al (1997) as being:

▶ The existence of a tradition and culture that discourages the open expression of emotion.

▶ The perception of clinical supervision as a management monitoring tool.

▶ The perception of clinical supervision as a form of personal therapy.

▶ A continuing lack of clarity regarding the purpose of supervision.

▶ Resistance itself being a component of any change process.

It is acknowledged that significant barriers exist preventing the widespread implementation of clinical supervision into modern nursing practice. It is hoped that the content of this book will give you information, assistance and very practical advice in creating for yourself a working and healthy clinical supervision culture where you work.

REFERENCES

Agnew, T. (1998) DoH holds back new figures on shortages. *Nursing Standard*; 12: 26, 5.

Butterworth, C.A. (1993) *Delphi Study of Optimum Practice in Nursing, Midwifery and Health Visiting*. Manchester: University of Manchester.

Clothier, C., MacDonald, C.A., Shaw, D.A. (1994) *The Allitt Enquiry*. London: HMSO.

Department of Health (1993) *A Vision for the Future: The Nursing, Midwifery and Health Visiting Contribution to Health and Healthcare*. London: HMSO.

Faugier, J., Butterworth, C.A. (1993) *Position Paper on Clinical Supervision*. Manchester: University of Manchester.

Haddock, J., Bassett, C. (1997) Nurses' perceptions of reflective practice. *Nursing Standard*; 11: 32, 39–41.

Lipley, N., Stokes, B. (1998) A real solution to nursing shortages? *Nursing Standard*; 12: 34, 12–13.

Middleman, R., Rhodes, G. (1985) *Competent Supervision: Making Imaginative Judgements*. Englewood Cliffs, NJ: Prentice Hall.

United Kingdom Central Council for Nursing, Midwifery and Health Visiting (1994) *Post Registration Education and Practice Project*. London: UKCC.

United Kingdom Central Council for Nursing, Midwifery and Health Visiting (1995) *Position Statement on Clinical Supervision for Nursing and Health Visiting*. London: UKCC.

United Kingdom Central Council for Nursing, Midwifery and Health Visiting (1996) *Further Guidance on Clinical Supervision for Nursing and Health Visiting*. London: UKCC.

Wilkin, P., Bowers, L., Monk, J. (1997) Clinical supervision: managing the resistance. *Nursing Times*; 93: 8, 48–49.

2 The benefits of clinical supervision

Nicola Clibbens

The benefits of clinical supervision are proposed in much of the nursing literature in this field (Butterworth and Faugier, 1992; Lowry, 1998; Mahood et al, 1998) and recent studies have aimed to measure the outcomes of clinical supervision (Butterworth, 1997). These attempts to measure the outcomes of clinical supervision are fraught with difficulty. Studies tend to focus on indicators such as 'job satisfaction', 'motivation' or 'stress and burnout' (Butterworth et al, 1997). These aspects of any given nurse's functioning are complex and are not influenced by clinical supervision in isolation. Taking job satisfaction as an example of this, factors such as a place on a course, a new ward manager or having a good holiday could have a positive effect on job satisfaction (Fig 2.1). Clinical supervision is therefore only one variable in this measure. It is a question of attribution. Changes in levels of job satisfaction cannot be attributed solely to the use of clinical supervision.

The drive to measure the positive effects of clinical supervision is, in part, a response to the cost of its implementation in health services. It is important to establish the benefits in order that nursing can put forward a clear case that the value of clinical supervision outweighs the cost in resources. A key reason for measuring these benefits is also to establish the outcome for patients. One could argue that by establishing the ways in which nurses benefit from clinical supervision, the benefits to patients become clearer. It is the assumption that the patient is at the core of clinical

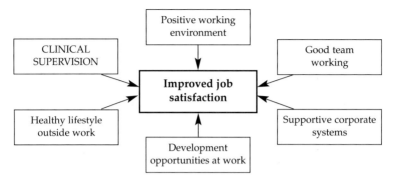

Fig 2.1 The factors which influence nurses' levels of job satisfaction

supervision. By helping nurses to grow personally and professionally the patients will ultimately benefit. The drive to establish the benefits or outcomes of clinical supervision in nursing remains, therefore, an important area of inquiry.

It is suggested in much of the recent nursing literature that clinical supervision will tackle a multitude of problems faced by nurses. Goorapah (1997) suggests that clinical supervision is too readily assumed to be the panacea for nursing, offering assistance in a wide spectrum of areas, such as management, education, clinical practice, patient care, support, professional growth, self and morale. Carthy (1994) expresses concern that if too much is expected from clinical supervision, the outcome may be disappointing. From my own supervisory practice, nurses do experience benefits in many ways. It could be argued that it is the anticipation of these benefits that motivates nurses to utilise clinical supervision to its full potential. It would, however, be unrealistic to expect that all nurses experience benefits in all these areas all of the time. The nature of clinical supervision is such that the supervisee will experience different benefits at different times, depending on the issues in their practice at that time.

Tim's story

Tim has worked in acute surgery for six months following registration and the remainder of his experience is in acute medicine. He has been a senior staff nurse in acute medicine for the past four years. He has been successful at interview for a post as senior staff nurse in the intensive care unit of the same hospital.

Tim has received clinical supervision every two months for the past year. He has elected to continue with the same clinical supervisor.

Tim's level of expertise in acute medical nursing is high. He is able to work with a high degree of perceptual accuracy; that is to say that he is at expert level in his practice. Expert practitioners are able to make highly perceptive and analytical clinical assessments, moving directly to the heart of the problem rather than relying on process or structure. Tim's needs in clinical supervision were to review critical incidents where he had dealt with highly complex situations. Tim would question the overriding principles of practice and he would function in the realm of generating new knowledge through reflection.

Having taken up his post in intensive care, Tim expressed a high level of anxiety and frustration. He was no longer an expert; he possessed many of the skills required to carry out his role but felt he was not as able as some

		Tim in acute medicine	Tim in intensive care
1	Novice		
2	Advanced beginner		
3	Competent		**Clinical supervision needs** Work through anxieties Work through the process of change Explore decision-making
4	Proficient		
5	Expert	**Clinical supervision needs** Critical incidents Analyse broad principles applied to practice Develop new knowledge	

(Benner, 1984)

Fig 2.2 Benefits derived from clinical supervision vary depending on the nurse's clinical practice at any given time

of his colleagues. The competent practitioner is one who is able to carry out the tasks required in caring for patients but lacks the ability to plan ahead and work in a rapidly flexible way. Problems require some analytical contemplation before a solution can be found. Tim's needs in his clinical supervision had changed – he needed to review his performance and explore his time management in intensive care nursing. Tim shared his decision-making problems and explored alternative actions (Fig 2.2).

The benefits of clinical supervision for Tim will be very different in his new role. He is more likely to benefit from the restorative aspects of supervision which acknowledge that nursing is stressful. He is most likely to use his clinical supervision to explore his clinical decision-making and look for alternative ways forward. One of the benefits that Tim will experience is from having developed his skills as a supervisee. He is much more likely to be able to utilise his clinical supervision in a purposeful way, taking a lead in the direction of sessions. This skilled use of clinical supervision will enable his development in his new post and build his confidence as a nurse in intensive care.

Supervisees benefit from clinical supervision in different ways at different times depending on the issues in their clinical practice at any given time. The benefits of clinical supervision are wider than just those that affect the individual nurse. The benefits can be described in three realms:

▶ Personal benefits – where the individual grows personally and professionally.

▶ Professional benefits – where the profession as a whole grows and develops.

▶ Organisational benefits – where organisations such as healthcare trusts and the independent sector benefit as a result of clinical supervision.

The focus of this chapter will be the benefits of clinical supervision to individual nurses. It is important, however, to briefly consider the benefits of clinical supervision to the profession and to the wider organisation of healthcare.

Clinical supervision is an issue for the whole profession of nursing. Although it is not a statutory requirement in nursing, unlike midwifery, it is increasingly an expectation that nurses will take an active part in clinical supervision (UKCC, 1996). Butterworth and Faugier (1992) view clinical supervision as the vehicle by which nurses can move from a position of oppressed underdog to one of increased autonomy and emancipation as professionals.

The increased autonomy of nurses goes hand in hand with the developing awareness in nursing of the implications of accountability. Clinical supervision is an ideal venue for individual nurses to explore their accountability in relation to clinical practice. The wider implication is the development of a system that further aids the development of knowledge unique to nursing. Nurses are enabled to explore the nature of nursing and their roles, thereby becoming more able to express clear notions of the nature of nursing.

Nursing is increasingly recognised as a profession with regulatory bodies and a code of conduct (UKCC, 1992). Clinical supervision is, at least in part, a means to ensure that standards of practice are in accordance with the code of conduct (UKCC, 1992). It could be argued that this is not the key aim of clinical supervision and that the essence of clinical supervision is not to act as a watchdog for clinical practice. Darley (1996) shares his concerns that clinical supervision is an ineffective method for the management of risks and that existing management systems are more effective means to ensure that clinical practice remains within safe boundaries. Equally, it could be argued that to assume that clinical supervision is the watchdog for clinical practice is a limited view of the potential benefit of clinical supervision. Clinical supervision is capable of developing practice to new standards rather than maintaining the status quo.

It has been proposed in much of the nursing literature that clinical supervision reduces stress in the nursing workforce. It is anticipated by many healthcare organisations that this will result in reduced sickness and absence. It is, however, doubtful that any healthcare organisations have been able to identify reduced sickness and absence thus far. Even if this effect were noted, it is subject to many other influences, not only clinical supervision.

A more realistic expectation is perhaps the beneficial effect the implementation of clinical supervision can have on recruitment of nurses. In an era where the nursing workforce cannot meet the health demands of the population in Britain, organisations where clinical supervision is offered are more likely to attract motivated nursing staff. Again it has been postulated that the retention of staff is more likely in organisations where clinical supervision is an accepted norm of practice. It is equally difficult to measure this effect and there are no studies currently which have identified this benefit.

Proctor's (1986) model divides clinical supervision into three main function groups: normative, formative and restorative. The application of Proctor's model in this way enables exploration of the benefits of clinical supervision for individual nurses. The use of Proctor's theory in action in supervisory practice helps to illuminate the theory as applied to practice. Butterworth et al (1997) explain the three functions of supervision proposed by Proctor as:

▶ Normative – which takes into account the quality control aspects of practice.

▶ Formative – which is linked to education and reflection.

▶ Restorative – which recognises emotional stress.

The model proposed by Proctor was not intended to be dissected into its component parts and I would argue strongly that in every exchange in clinical supervision all three functions exist. For ease of explanation, however, specific examples from supervisory practice will be explained in terms of the realm that is most dominant in that instance.

THE NORMATIVE FUNCTION

The normative function of clinical supervision, in my experience, is met with a degree of suspicion among novice supervisors and supervisees. At first glance it appears to fulfil the notion of management control and 'big brother' keeping practice in line with policy. While this suspicion is unfounded to a great extent, it is true to assume that there is an element of supervision which is about ensuring that practice is of an acceptable quality and meets local and national policy and guidelines. My approach to those who doubt the value of this function in clinical supervision is twofold. First, one cannot expect clinical supervision to be of benefit without a degree of challenge (Bond and Holland, 1998). Some of the challenge will come from exploring the boundaries of practice and issues of quality in clinical practice. Second, I feel that the normative function of clinical supervision is the safety net guarding against unsafe practice. Clinical supervision is a place where real issues of clinical practice can be shared and risks managed through the exploration of appropriate clinical practices and resolution for difficult problems. There are limitations, however, to the extent to which clinical supervision can be assumed to manage clinical risks (Darley, 1996). The supervisor has to rely on the supervisee's reports of their clinical practice and can only assume that they have given an accurate interpretation of reality. Therefore, the supervisor has limited ability to objectively understand the practice of the supervisee and relies on subjective reporting.

It is an expectation of the nature of the relationship in clinical supervision that the exploration of normative issues will be based on the supervisee 'doing it themselves' and not 'having it done to them'. That is, the supervisee examines the quality of their *own* work against agreed standards rather than the supervisor giving feedback on their performance. This subtle but important distinction is one of the ways in which clinical supervision differs in emphasis from appraisal systems.

James' story

James expressed concern regarding the level of accountability that can be taken by student nurses who are on rostered service placements prior to registration on the UKCC professional register.

His main concerns were whether they could be allowed to carry out an admission procedure without a registered nurse present.

The issues were explored by brainstorming the possible reasons why student nurses should or should not carry out the admission procedure unobserved. These were formulated into a list in order to clarify thinking on the issue (Fig 2.3). Using pen and paper to make notes as you talk can help to add focus to the session and give both the supervisor and the supervisee a point of reference. The list then becomes an *aide-mémoire*

Should do admissions	Should not do admissions
• Gives them the opportunity to practise their skills.	• How can the students' skills be assessed if the RN never sees their work?
• Will be expected to do it in a matter of weeks anyway.	• Should patients be given a choice?
• Cannot expect the development of skills if prevented from doing it.	• Are there any standards that state that all patients must be seen by a registered nurse on arrival in hospital?
• Do not have the resources to ensure that rostered students are always supervised by a registered nurse (they are in the numbers in the off duty).	• Are students equipped to deal with difficult situations that could arise during the admission procedure?
• Custom and practice – rostered students have always done admissions.	• Where does the RN stand in terms of their accountability for the wellbeing of the patient?

Fig 2.3 Brainstorm of whether student nurses should carry out the admission procedure unobserved

throughout the session. In this session no solutions were found but the supervisee left with a clearer notion of the key issues. The supervisee decided to compare and analyse the issues with local and national policy and use this as the method of decision-making, as suggested in the normative aspect of Proctor's (1986) model.

The benefit to the supervisee was to gain clarity of thought around a problem that appeared hazy and vague at first (Bond and Holland, 1998). The supervisee was able to work through each issue logically as it occurred to him and add it to a logical set of ideas in the form of a list. In this example it was not possible to apply the ideas to policy or standards in the session, as neither the supervisor nor the supervisee were clear which documents were relevant. It is appropriate in this instance to encourage the supervisee to continue to work on the issue outside the supervision session.

THE FORMATIVE FUNCTION

Clinical supervision supports learning in the individual. The process of learning occurs in many different ways and cannot always be adequately described by reducing the experience down to concrete examples. Supervisees learn in ways that are reflective and very individual to them. Reflection is an integral part of clinical supervision and occurs through open questioning by the supervisor, who guides the supervisee throughout the problem (Johns, 1995). The supervisor deals with the issues brought by the supervisee and prompts and encourages review of the events as they are presented. The supervisee is helped to use knowledge and imagination to examine problems and illuminate the way forward. One of the benefits of clinical supervision identified in a study by Wright et al (1997) is 'reflecting on solutions in clinical practice and how these have been handled'.

Gloria's story

Gloria has just qualified as a mental health nurse. She expressed her frustration at her inability to fully utilise therapeutic interventions with clients due to the pressure of work on a busy acute ward. She wanted to explore new ways of working therapeutically within the constraints of the ward environment.

Gloria was encouraged to explore the care of a specific client in more detail. She brainstormed possible therapeutic approaches and discussed the relative pros and cons for each. Having reviewed her options, the sticking point for Gloria was a feeling that she never had time to do anything. She was encouraged to review the structure and activity during a typical day. She then moved forward to identify the activities that she could change. By the end of the session Gloria had reviewed her options and critically reviewed her time management skills in relation to therapeutic interventions.

In this example there are benefits for Gloria in all three functions of clinical supervision (Proctor, 1986). Focusing on the formative benefits, however, Gloria was facilitated in reflecting on her situation and the care of patients. It is evident that as she went through the process of recounting her situation in a calm and safe way, new ideas and solutions started to appear to her with little prompting. Gloria had been challenged to think about her time management. She was able to identify times when she could implement the therapeutic interventions she wanted to use and felt that she would be able to try to change her practice. She had also explored subtle modifications to the therapy to enable positive outcomes in a ward environment, which still met the needs of the client. The learning that had taken place was complex; the supervisee knew which therapeutic interventions were appropriate to meet the clients' needs but was unable to apply them in the ward environment. Through the process of reflection and problem solving, the supervisee was able to take her practice forward by finding imaginative ways of working.

The wellbeing of the client is at the heart of clinical supervision and clinical supervision should focus on clinical practice (UKCC, 1996). Supervisors, however, need to take the widest view of the component parts of clinical practice. The supervisee's learning needs may appear to be at the periphery of clinical work and yet may be crucial to the development of that nurse. Some of the benefits of clinical supervision reported by nurses include 'improving professional development processes' and 'identifying skills they possess or need' (Kohner, 1994).

Jane's story

Jane had arranged her own clinical supervision and had met with her clinical supervisor seven times. She shared with her supervisor that she had experienced difficulty when asked to deliver a presentation. This was a key issue for her because she intended applying for promotion to ward sister and the selection process included a short presentation.

The approach to the formative aspect of clinical supervision for Jane was much more specific and practical. Beginning with some exploratory work, Jane reviewed previous experiences of presentations and where she felt her strengths and weaknesses lay. She agreed to take a goal-directed approach where homework was carried out between sessions. Having spent several sessions reviewing literature regarding presentation skills, Jane prepared an outline for a presentation and explored the practical issues around its delivery with her supervisor. Eventually Jane used the work she had done in supervision to present to her colleagues, who evaluated her performance. Jane used the evaluations as the basis for one of her sessions.

The supervisee has developed a new skill through the process of clinical supervision. It could be argued that presentation skills are peripheral to clinical care but, in this example, I would suggest that the supervisee has increased her confidence in skills that can be applied to many areas of nursing. The supervisee is able to identify situations, such as hand over, case reviews, team meetings and clinical teaching sessions, where she feels much more self-assured.

Some aspects of learning that occur in clinical supervision are less tangible. The very fact that the supervisee has been part of a supervisory relationship equips them to become effective clinical supervisors themselves. The nature of the processes and relationships that occur in clinical supervision will have been explored in the live situation. From a more pragmatic stance, support can be offered to the supervisee in direct response to their developing role as a clinical supervisor themselves.

The nature of the relationship in clinical supervision has parallels with the relationship that nurses form with patients/clients. The skills adopted by the supervisor will have similarities to those used in the care of patients (Hawkins and Shohet, 1989). The supervisee can utilise the supervisory relationship to develop their interpersonal skills in clinical practice. This process occurs in two ways. First, the supervisee may raise the issue of interpersonal relationships for open discussion. In this way the sharing of ideas and solutions to problems is a learning experience for the supervisee. Second, and less tangible, the student will absorb the experiences of clinical supervision through processes such as role modelling and experiential learning. This process emphasises the need for nurses to have positive experiences of clinical supervision from skilled supervisors.

The supervisee clearly derives some benefits from clinical supervision in the formative function, but it should not be forgotten that the supervisor can gain a great deal from the verbal exchanges they have with their supervisees (Lowry, 1998). The clinical issues brought by the supervisee can often illuminate issues for the supervisor and the generation of ideas in the supervisor can be sparked off by the contribution of the supervisee. The key benefit to the supervisor is the continual development of their relationship building and facilitation skills. It is crucial, however, that the supervisor has the opportunity to explore their own issues in their own clinical supervision.

THE RESTORATIVE FUNCTION

The restorative function of clinical supervision can be viewed as a healing process. Nurses are in daily contact with emotional dependence, pain, confusion, illness, grief and death (Lowry, 1998). The pain and stress for nurses involved in carrying out these day-to-day activities is often unacknowledged. The restorative effects of clinical supervision occur in every encounter; one tends to fall back on the old adage, 'a problem shared is a problem halved'. The process of sharing and relationship building in clinical supervision is in itself a positive stress-relieving process. Attempts to quantify the stress-relieving benefits of clinical supervision have varied in their findings. Butterworth et al (1997) found that stress scores and burnout scores in nurses reduced slightly with the implementation of clinical supervision. This study found, however, that in some cases there was no significant change in stress or burnout. Despite this, the nursing literature continues to propose reduced stress levels as one of the key benefits of clinical supervision. Kohner (1994) found that nurses felt that clinical supervision 'provides acknowledgement of their stress and heavy workload' and Severinsson and Borgenhammar (1997) found that experts in nursing felt that clinical supervision prevents burnout and reduces stress by clarifying nurses' job function. It is my experience that the act of sharing problems faced in everyday clinical practice has immediate visible stress-lifting effects on the supervisee. At its most basic level, being heard relieves stress. The stress-relieving benefits of clinical supervision are increased by the skilled exploration of the problem by the supervisor. Stress is reduced in the supervisee even when solutions or answers to the problem are not found. The act of sharing appears to have a profound effect on the supervisee's ability to cope with the everyday stresses of being a nurse.

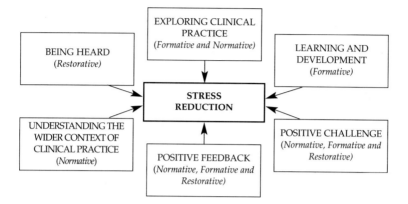

Fig 2.4 The aspects of clinical supervision that can relieve stress

The restorative aspect of clinical supervision is evident in every supervisory contact; it is at the core of every interaction. Taking the three functions of clinical supervision proposed by Proctor (1986) it can be argued that the formative and normative functions are stress-relieving and complement the restorative function rather than being distinct and separate functions (Fig 2.4).

The work of Hawkins and Shohet (1989) focuses on the notion that nurses are 'wounded helpers'. These wounds result from the stresses faced by nurses who care for people in difficult circumstances. It is proposed that these wounds can have a positive influence on our understanding of the suffering of others and therefore promote the use of empathic responses. One could equally argue that it is these wounds which prevent nurses from maintaining their humanity, empathy and energy for caring (Bond and Holland, 1998). The continued development of self-awareness can help nurses to ensure that their wounds do not prevent caring relationships from being developed in clinical practice.

Clinical supervision can facilitate the exploration of the self, leading to positive outcomes for the supervisee and the patients for whom they care (Bond and Holland, 1998). The development of self occurs when the supervisee is given the opportunity to stand back from their clinical practice and observe the processes which they use, rather like a fly on the wall, looking down at your own practice. The use of frameworks of reflection can support this process, such as Johns' model (Fig 2.5).

Aesthetics	• What was I trying to achieve? • Why did I respond as I did? • What were the consequences of my actions • How was this person/persons feeling? • How did I know this?
Personal	• How did I feel in this situation? • What internal factors were influencing me?
Ethics	• How did my actions match my beliefs? • What factors made me act in incongruent ways?
Reflexivity	• How does this connect with previous experiences? • Could I handle this better in similar situations? • What would be the consequences of alternative actions? • How did I feel about this experience? • Can I support myself and others as a consequence? • Has this changed my way of knowing?

(Johns, 1995)

Fig 2.5 Johns' model of structured reflection

It is my experience that this aspect of clinical supervision causes a great deal of anxiety among novice supervisors in nursing. Nurses express concern that they do not possess the skills required to facilitate this level of exploration of practice. Nurses often feel that they would need to be qualified counsellors to take on this depth of analysis of self and clinical practice. This is a key issue for the establishment of clinical supervision in nursing that is of benefit to nurses. The UKCC (1996) clearly states that clinical supervisors should have training before acting as a clinical supervisor. While it is unrealistic to suggest that nurses should be trained in counselling skills before acting as clinical supervisors, training should cover issues that begin the process of development of these skills.

It is a valid fear that supervisors attempting to pursue deeper levels of analysis of practice without adequate experience or skills could potentially be damaging to supervisees. There are safeguards in the process of supervision that should always be utilised to avoid negative experiences of clinical supervision. The process of developing ground rules, often referred to as a contract, should cover issues such as the supervisor's level of skill and expertise in clinical supervision (Mahood et al, 1998). The depth reached in clinical supervision should match the expertise of the supervisor in order for the process to remain safe and beneficial to the supervisee. The supervisor should always receive clinical supervision. It is through the process of receiving clinical supervision and offering clinical supervision to others that supervisory skills are developed.

Gordon's story

Gordon has been a registered nurse for 18 months. He is keen to apply for a senior staff nurse post. He has difficulty thinking about his skills and appears to be quite negative about the contribution he can make to nursing.

Gordon began his supervision session by discussing his desire to apply for a senior staff nurse post. He was unable to clearly express his nursing skills. He appeared flat and deflated despite his obvious motivation to develop his career. Open questioning led to the development of a plan for the session. Gordon wanted to formulate clearer notions of where he was at in his career as a nurse. At first he simply talked through the issues which were uppermost for him.

The supervisor found it difficult to focus on key ideas and emphasise important points as he randomly talked through his thoughts. In these situations a degree of structure can help add logic and coherence to the supervisee's thoughts. It would have been appropriate to utilise a reflective model such as Johns' (1995) but in this session a SWOT analysis was used. This method was chosen in order to explicitly record the areas where Gordon had strengths, weaknesses, opportunities and threats in his career. This enabled Gordon to plan writing his CV and prepare for the interview. This process also encouraged Gordon to reflect on his skills and record his strengths, resulting in an increased feeling of self-confidence. Recording his weaknesses was equally as important as recording his strengths. His perceived weaknesses are likely to be a source of stress. This area was explored and gently challenged and ways to develop his skills were discussed. The discussion of opportunities and threats in his career helped Gordon to see himself in the wider context of the changing environment of healthcare and therefore make long and short term plans for the future.

The benefits of clinical supervision are broad and varied depending on the needs of the supervisee and the skills of the supervisor. The experiences of the supervisees explored in this chapter begin to illustrate the vast array of potential benefits of clinical supervision and also highlight the difficulty in measuring these benefits. It could be argued that the benefits are highly personal to the individual supervisee and at a level that is not always concrete and therefore not easily identified.

GROUP SUPERVISION

It is important to ensure that the model of supervision chosen in any given healthcare environment will reap the greatest possible benefit to the nursing team. The examples explored thus far focus on individual, one-to-one supervision. Supervision in groups, teams and networks can be beneficial and should be chosen because of the benefits, rather than as a cost-effective method of supervising more than one person at a time.

Group supervision can benefit its members by the dynamic nature of group processes in the generation of ideas. Ideas developed in a group have a quality that is unique to group working, often referred to as 'synergism' (Kitzinger, 1994). This is where the putting together of many minds can generate new ideas that could not have been developed between two people. This applies to resolution to clinical problems as well as the generation of ideas. Many different solutions are likely to be found in a group, and solutions will be found that have been created by the group which no individual in the group would have generated on their own. Group supervision, therefore, allows for a greater scope of experience to be shared (Bond and Holland, 1998).

One of the benefits of group or team supervision is the shared understanding of roles, responsibilities and working styles. Team supervision can aid the development of team working. The supervisees would be enabled to explore their responses to each other in the team and in clinical practice. This enables a deeper understanding in the individual of the effects of their own contribution to the team.

The benefits of group and team clinical supervision can only be achieved when a skilled supervisor leads the way and ensures safety for the group. Ideally, the supervisor would possess group facilitation skills and an understanding of the dynamics of groups. It is important to consider the limitations of group supervision. It will not be of benefit to all nurses; some individuals find sharing in groups very difficult and are inhibited by group members who are more confident. Some issues for nurses are difficult to share in a group, which is a more public arena than individual supervision. It may be appropriate to offer a variety of models of supervision in order that the nurses themselves can use the model that meets their needs most effectively.

REFERENCES

Benner, P. (1984) *From Novice to Expert: Excellence and Power in Clinical Nursing Practice.* Menlo Park, California: Addison-Wesley Publishing.

Bond, M., Holland, S. (eds.) (1998) *Skills of Clinical Supervision for Nurses.* Buckingham: Open University Press.

Butterworth, T., Carson, J., White, E. et al (1997) *It's Good to Talk: Clinical Supervision and Mentorship. An Evaluation Study in England and Scotland.* Manchester: University of Manchester.

Butterworth, T., Faugier, J. (eds.) (1992) *Clinical Supervision and Mentorship in Nursing.* London: Chapman and Hall.

Carthy, J. (1994) Bandwagons Roll. *Nursing Standard*; 8: 38, 3.

Darley, M. (1996) Can clinical supervision improve risk management? *Health Care Risk Report*; March 1996, 20–21.

Goorapah, D. (1997) Clinical supervision. *Journal of Clinical Nursing*; 6, 173–178.

Hawkins, P., Shohet, R. (1989) *Supervision in the Helping Professions.* Milton Keynes: Open University Press.

Johns, C. (1995) Framing learning through reflection within Carper's fundamental ways of knowing in nursing. *Journal of Advanced Nursing*; 22, 22.

Kitzinger, J. (1994) The methodology of focus groups: the importance of interaction between participants. *Sociology of Health and Illness*; 16: 1, 103–121.

Kohner, N. (1994) *Clinical Supervision in Practice.* London: King's Fund Centre.

Lowry, M. (1998) Clinical supervision for the development of nursing practice. *British Journal of Nursing*; 7: 9, 553–558.

Mahood, N., McFadden, K., Colgan, L. et al (1998) Clinical supervision: the Cartmel NDU experience. *Nursing Standard*; 12: 26, 44–47.

Proctor, B. (1986) Supervision: a co-operative exercise in accountability. In: Marken, M., Payne, M. (eds.) *Enabling and Ensuring.* Leicester: Leicester National Youth Bureau and Council for Education and Training in Youth and Community Work.

Severinsson, E.I., Borgenhammar, E.V. (1997) Expert views on clinical supervision: a study based on interviews. *Journal of Nursing Management;* 5, 175–183.

United Kingdom Central Council for Nursing, Midwifery and Health Visiting (1992) *Code of Professional Conduct.* (3rd edition) London: UKCC.

United Kingdom Central Council for Nursing, Midwifery and Health Visiting (1996) *Position Statement on Clinical Supervision for Nursing and Health Visiting.* London: UKCC.

Wright, S., Elliott, M., Schofield, H. (1997) A networking approach to clinical supervision. *Nursing Standard;* 11: 18, 39–41.

FURTHER READING

Marrow, C.E., Macauley, D.M., Crumbie, A. (1997) Promoting reflective practice through structured clinical supervision. *Journal of Nursing Management;* 5, 77–82.

3 Models of supervision

Deborah Glover

First the bad news. This chapter will not give you a definitive model of supervision to use in your organisation. 'But this is why I'm reading this chapter,' I hear you cry. But stop for a moment to consider the models used within nursing so far. For example, those that were supposed to help us plan, implement and evaluate nursing care, such as Roper, Logan and Tierny (1985), Roy (1984) and Neuman (1982). How successful were they when 'rolled out' to every ward, department and health centre? How often were you left trying to fit your particular patients' problems and needs into one of these models and wondering what to do with the left over bits – those that didn't slot into any of the categories?

Well, it's a bit like that with supervision. Unfortunately, there are numerous models described by numerous authors: Bishop (1998), Butterworth (1998), Fowler (1996) and Nicklin (1997) to name but a few. Given the diversity of cultures and organisational structures within the NHS and healthcare generally, and the fact that each nurse will have their own needs and requirements from the supervision process, to suggest any one model would be pure folly. What works well in midwifery will not necessarily work in psychiatry and what works in psychiatry may not work in health visiting. It would be almost impossible to use a 'prescribed' model for your requirements and think it will be all things to all people. Chances are you will need to mix and match two or three models then 'suck it and see', making any necessary adjustments until it is right for you.

Faugier and Butterworth (1994), however, state that models fall into three categories:

▶ Models which describe the supervision in relation to the supervisory relationship and its main functions.

▶ Models which describe the elements of the main functions of supervision.

▶ Development models which look closely at the process of the supervisory relationship.

I would suggest that just choosing a model on the basis of one of the above is just as limiting as choosing one just because you can pronounce the name of the author. Consider each of the elements of the above and the points outlined below.

POINTS TO CONSIDER

Before deciding on which model, or which components of models, you may wish to explore, it is useful to explore what you and your team consider to be the main functions and benefits of supervision and what you want to get out of it. Once these have been decided and agreed, you can adapt you model to incorporate these elements.

A definition

This is vital. There are as many definitions as there are people who will tell you they can define supervision. Here are just a few:

'A formal arrangement that enables nurses, midwives and health visitors to discuss their work regularly with another experienced professional. Clinical supervision involves reflecting on practice in order to learn from experience and improve competence.' (Kohner, 1994)

'A term used to describe a formal process of professional support and learning which enables individual practitioners to develop knowledge and competence, assume responsibility for their own practice and enhance consumer protection and safety of care in complex clinical situations. It is central to the process of learning and to the scope of professional practice and should be seen as a means of encouraging self-assessment and analytical and reflective skills.' (Department of Health, 1993)

'A designated interaction between two or more practitioners, within a safe and supportive environment, which enables a continuum of reflective, critical analysis of care, to ensure quality patient services.' (Bishop, 1998)

All illustrate the different ways that the nature and purpose of supervision is viewed. However, any definition that has an underpinning philosophy of support and development for staff should be viewed favourably.

It might be worth mentioning here what clinical supervision *is not*.

'It is not a managerial control system; therefore clinical supervision is not the exercise of overt managerial responsibility or managerial supervision, not a system of formal individual performance review, nor hierarchical in nature.' (UKCC, 1996)

The UKCC does go on to say that 'links between clinical supervision and management are important. These links are best described in the local policy and ground rules. Management may wish to evaluate the impact of supervision and its service benefits. Development and establishment of clinical supervision should, therefore, involve managers and practitioners with the emphasis on a 'light touch' management influence.' (UKCC, 1996)

The principles of supervision

▶ Nursing skills should be constantly redefined and improved throughout one's professional life.

▶ Critical debate about professional activity is a means to professional development.

▶ Supervision should begin with professional education and continue thereafter as an integral part of professional development.

▶ It is not an incidental event and requires time and energy.

▶ Organisational commitment is stated.

(Butterworth, 1998 – although he defines these as 'ground rules'.)

These principles, especially the latter two, should be taken into account when considering a model. Supervision doesn't come cheap and you will need to demonstrate to the stakeholders in the organisation the cost-benefit of it in order to gain commitment. Wolsey and Leach (1997) argue that you will need to demonstrate to these stakeholders that not only does it benefit you and your patients and that things will get a lot worse if supervision is lost, but also that there is a wider organisational benefit. Additionally, participants need to contribute time and energy to it. Therefore, a model that enables supervision to occur in the most efficient and effective way is crucial.

The aims of supervision

▶ To expand the knowledge base of practitioners (through guided reflection and sharing of knowledge, expertise and experience).

▶ To assist in developing professional proficiency.

▶ To develop the autonomy and self-esteem of the practitioner (Platt-Koch, 1986).

The functions of supervision

Supervision can be seen as having three main functions, as described by Proctor (1986):

▶ Formative (educational) function, which is related to developing knowledge, skills, research awareness and understanding in the supervisee. This is done through problem solving, the supervisor sharing knowledge and expertise, reflection, identifying training needs and exploring other perspectives.

▶ Restorative (supportive) function, which is support and counselling through the therapeutic supervision relationship which nurtures and cares for the supervisee. This is achieved through debriefing, feedback about practice, communication and support. It facilitates self-awareness through critical analysis and exploration of events and feelings.

▶ Normative function, related to the management aspect of the practitioner's role, such as maintaining standards and monitoring of quality. A word of caution here: Platt-Koch (1986) suggested that as this function provides the more managerial focus, there may be a danger that this will be confused with other managerial issues not directly connected with the issues raised in the supervision session.

Ground rules

The model should incorporate any ground rules you may wish to lay down for supervision sessions. Rules such as the frequency and length of meetings, the nature and boundaries of the relationship, along with the practicalities, such as where it will take place and how supervision can be integrated into existing work, should help to develop the model (Pritchard, 1997).

REFLECTION IN SUPERVISION

I have to admit I am a big fan of reflection within supervision, or indeed using a reflective model of supervision. It provides a valuable learning tool. So why do we need to reflect on our practice? Well, everyday nursing provides us with situations that are complex and often uncertain. In many instances, we cannot just apply theory or techno-rational approaches to the problem. Nursing is not just a series of simple decision-making steps and practice is, in part, based on previous experiences interacting with a particular situation.

Many practitioners will argue that they reflect on their practice anyway. However, often this is done in a haphazard, unstructured way. For example, there are some days we finish our shift and think to ourselves how awful it has been. The cancelled operation, snapping at the student nurse and knowing that Mr Smith obviously wasn't really happy when you walked away from him. The reflection on this will probably only take place on a superficial level and what with being busy and tomorrow being another day, the thoughts tend to be forgotten until a similar incident occurs.

Structured reflection, however, provides a framework with which to work through a problem or incident, considering possible influencing factors, and then use this information to explore alternative actions and their possible conclusions. This gives us insight and understanding and a new perspective for future reference.

What is reflective practice/learning?

Reflective learning can be defined as:

'A process of internally examining and exploring an issue of concern, triggered by an experience, which creates and clarifies meaning in terms of self, and which results in a changed conceptual perspective.' (Boyd and Fales (1983) cited in Atkins and Murphy, 1993)

In a paper presented at the First Reflective Practice Conference in Luton, England, Johns (1994a) stated that:

'Reflecting on experience enables the practitioner to assess his or her work experiences in order to explore, understand and develop the meaning of practice and to expose the contradictions between what he or she aims to achieve and the way he or she practices.'

And doesn't that just sum up what we are essentially trying to do when, as outlined above, we think about our day and why we didn't feel entirely happy with the way it had gone? But so often, as we do not reflect in a structured way, we are not able to explore and understand the meaning of practice, nor explore the contradictions between aim and achievement.

Johns goes on to say:

'Through this understanding and the conflict of contradiction, the practitioner can become empowered to take action to confront and resolve the contradictions towards achieving more desirable, more effective and more satisfying work.' (Johns, 1994b)

Schon (1983) suggests a three-dimensional paradigm for reflection:

► Knowing in action – the practitioner's actions are spontaneous and their judgements are not thought about in advance. It is an action we know how to do as we have done it successfully in the past (Ford and Walsh, 1994).

► Reflection in action – if, when applying your knowledge in a situation, you find that there was an adverse result, you realise that this obviously wasn't sufficient. If you reflect on the concepts implicit in the action and the feelings that led to your particular actions, you then evaluate these actions and reconstruct them in further action (Harris, 1996).

▶ Reflection on action – here, in order to understand what happened in light of the outcome, you reflect on the situation through retrospective analysis and interpretation. You consider how the situation may have been managed differently, what the outcomes may have been if the alternative actions were taken, and identify what other knowledge may have been useful in the situation. Because this occurs after the event, your skills, knowledge and future practice are developed.

A model for reflection

One of the most comprehensive and user-friendly models of reflection is that proposed by Johns (1994c). The framework has been developed and used with practitioners and involves a series of questions which helps them consider their experience in a structured and meaningful way. The model suggests:

Write a description of the event.

Cue questions to aid your reflection:

▶ What was I trying to achieve?

▶ Why did I respond as I did?

▶ What were the consequences of that for

the patient?

others?

myself?

▶ How was this person(s) feeling?

▶ How did I know this?

▶ How did I feel in this situation?

▶ What internal factors were influencing me?

▶ How did my actions match my beliefs?

▶ What factors made me act in incongruent ways?

▶ What knowledge did or should inform me?

▶ How does this connect with my previous experience?

▶ Can I support myself and others as a consequence?

▶ Has this changed my way of knowing?

The degree to which one answers these questions, indeed the number that are asked of oneself, will vary from individual to individual. As Johns concludes:

'The type of knowledge developed through reflection is termed 'personal knowledge' – personal in the sense that it is unique to the practitioner and is contextual in response to the various clinical situations the practitioner is involved with. Reflection aims to develop the quantity and quality of the practitioner's repertoire of available skilled interventions and the quality of the practitioner's intuitive grasp and response.'

Reflection can, however, bring to the surface feelings or thoughts that may be uncomfortable for the practitioner. But if reflection is undertaken with the help and support of an experienced supervisor, these feelings can be explored in a logical and 'safe' way, the ultimate benefit being a confident, reflective practitioner who is open and willing to explore experiences in practice.

WAYS OF DOING IT

As well as considering the principle, aims, function and content of the supervision process, you also need to consider how you are actually going to do it and how often.

Clarke et al (1998), describe the use of 'structural' and 'process' models.

Structural models

One-to-one supervision

One supervisor and one supervisee. This can be either with a supervisor from your own discipline or with a supervisor from a different discipline.

Advantages

▶ Building a trusting relationship with the supervisor.

▶ You are more likely to attend sessions.

▶ 'Privacy' – this is especially useful for junior nurses who may not wish to 'open up' in front of colleagues.

▶ You will prepare for the session, as it is more personal to your needs and practice.

▶ Practical and easy to arrange.

▶ Continuity – the same supervisor every time.

Disadvantages

▶ Problems may occur if you do not like your supervisor.

▶ You don't get the benefit of other views and experiences.

▶ Time consuming for the supervisor, as they are likely to have more than one person to supervise.

▶ Expensive.

▶ Can become 'intense' – initially the supervisee may become very reliant on the supervisor and often will expect more of a 'counselling' relationship than a guiding one.

Group supervision

More than three people involved. The ideal maximum is six people who can be from different grades and clinical areas.

Advantages

▶ Supervisee benefits from the guidance and expertise of both the supervisor and the members of the group.

▶ It is more cost effective.

▶ Less emotionally 'intense' for the supervisor.

▶ You can build support and facilitative relationships with other group members.

▶ Group dynamics can be stimulating.

Disadvantages

▶ The group may take a long time to 'gel', thus the process and benefits take time to emerge.

▶ Members of the group and the supervisor have to contend with group dynamics.

▶ It can feel threatening for less experienced staff.

▶ It's easier to skip sessions if you know others will be there.

▶ High levels of skill are needed from the supervisor.

Triadic/consultative

Three people involved, although the interaction is essentially between the supervisor and the supervisee.

Advantages

▶ The 'extra' practitioner, usually a practice development nurse or clinical nurse specialist, adds an extra dimension to the discussion.

▶ The third party may also act as a coach enabling supervisor and supervisee to develop their skills.

Disadvantages

▶ Having an extra person involved may be threatening.

▶ They may not have the supervisory skills necessary.

Network

A group of practitioners from the same clinical area.

Advantages

▶ Group members are more likely to understand your particular issues as they can relate to that area of practice.

▶ Can discuss new developments.

Disadvantages

▶ May be 'insular', that is only focus on their speciality and don't consider the wider context.

▶ Difficult to organise.

Process models

Managerial

This has disadvantages and advantages. Having a manager as a supervisor can show the supervisee that the manager is committed to supervision and will therefore support it within the organisation. However, the major disadvantage is that at the end of the day, your manager will always have the authority to discipline you and they may find it difficult to separate their managerial/supervisory role. Therefore, are you likely to be as open and reflective about your practice in front of them? In some instances your manager may not be clinically involved on a day-to-day basis, so will they be able to give you expert guidance on clinical issues?

Peer

The main problem with peer supervision is the danger of becoming too 'cosy'. As peers, they will be aware of the issues you may be discussing and will therefore tend to be more supportive than challenging during the session, which means there will be less skills or personal development.

Non-managerial hierarchical

Here, it is hoped that the supervisor will be an expert in the area, with established supervisory skills. As they are not 'management' they are less threatening because they cannot discipline the supervisee. However, it must be remembered that if the supervisor is a nurse, they still have a duty under the Code of Professional Conduct (UKCC, 1992) to challenge poor or dangerous practice and, if necessary, report it.

Reflective model (Johns, 1996)

Reflection can be undertaken by the practitioner at any time, not just within the supervision session. It is a useful tool for both supervisor and supervisee to prepare for and structure the session. The supervisor can use their skills and experience in a more directive way.

CONCLUSION

Wolsey and Leach (1997) found that many supervision models have not yet been tested or verified empirically. Those that have, and have been found to be deficient, have not been modified and they are tied to models of counselling and therapy.

There are also some cynics who have suggested that there are two less favourable models of supervision. First, the Nominal Model, where supervision is seen as a necessary activity, but there are no resources or time in which to carry it out effectively, so its main purpose is to provide a façade that supervision is being practised. Second, the Prescriptive Model, based on the view that the supervisor needs to correct deficiencies in the practice of the supervisee and the primary purpose of the supervision is to correct those flaws.

To me, the ideal model is the Reflective Model, based on the notion that all nurses, whatever their grade or job, need skilled support to develop and refine their own efforts to improve practice. Its primary purpose is the stimulation of guided reflection based on the processes and outcomes of nursing.

The model chosen will ultimately depend on the emphasis you want to place on your supervision (Hawkins and Shohet, 1989) and what you want to achieve from it. You will need to consider:

- the needs of the practitioner;
- the purpose of clinical supervision;
- who will be the supervisor;
- the time involved;
- the work context.

(Clarke et al, 1998)

Fowler (1996) states that a model of supervision should address three areas. First, it should describe the role and function of supervision within the practice of nursing. Second, it should identify the constituents of the supervisory relationship. Third, it should describe the process of the relationship. Johns (1993) suggests that the model should also acknowledge the practical nature of nursing, so it would need to take into account the more mundane issues, such as how long it should take and where it should occur.

REFERENCES

Atkins, S., Murphy, K. (1993) Reflection: a review of the literature. *Journal of Advanced Nursing*; 18: 8, 1188–1192.

Bishop, V. (1998) Clinical supervision: what is it? In: Bishop, V. (ed.) *Clinical Supervision in Practice*. London: Macmillan/NT Research.

Butterworth, A. (1998) Clinical supervision as an emerging idea in nursing. In: Butterworth, A., Faugier, J., Burnard, P. (eds.) *Clinical Supervision and Mentorship in Nursing*. Cheltenham: Stanley Thornes.

Clarke, A., Dooher, J., Fowler, J. et al (1998) Implementing clinical supervision. In: Fowler, J. (ed.) *The Handbook of Clinical Supervision: Your Questions Answered*. Salisbury: Quay Books, Mark Allen Publishing.

Department of Health (1993) *A Vision for the Future: The Nursing, Midwifery and Health Visiting Contribution to Healthcare*. London: HMSO.

Faugier, J., Butterworth, A. (1994) *Clinical Supervision: A Position Paper*. Manchester: University of Manchester.

Ford, P., Walsh, M. (1994) *New Rituals for Old: Nursing Through the Looking Glass*. Oxford: Butterworth-Heinemann.

Fowler, J. (1996) The organisation of clinical supervision within the nursing profession: a review of the literature. *Journal of Advanced Nursing*; 23, 471–478.

Harris, M. (1996) Reflective learning as a strategy for enabling undergraduate nursing students. *Assignment – Ongoing Work of Health Care Students*; Vol. 2: No. 2.3, 2.4, August 1996–January 1997.

Hawkins, P., Shohet, R. (1989) *Supervision in the Helping Professions*. Milton Keynes: Open University Press.

Johns, C. (1993) Professional supervision. *Journal of Nursing Management*; 1, 9–18.

Johns, C. (1994a, b, c) *Significance of reflective practice for nursing practice.* Paper presented at the First Reflective Practice Conference – 'Learning Through Experience'. Luton: University of Luton.

Johns, C. (1996) The benefits of a reflective model of nursing. *Nursing Times*; 92: 40, 39–41.

Kohner, N. (1994) *Clinical Supervision in Practice.* London: King's Fund Centre.

Neuman, B. (1982) *The Neuman Systems Model: Application to Nursing, Education and Practice.* New York, NY: Appleton and Lange.

Nicklin, P. (1997) A practice-centred model of clinical supervision. *Nursing Times*; 93: 46, 52–54.

Platt-Koch, L. (1986) Clinical supervision for psychiatric nurses. *Journal of Psychosocial Nursing*; 26: 1, 6–15.

Pritchard, T. (1997) Supervision in practice. *Nursing in Critical Care*; 2: 1, 34–37.

Proctor, B. (1986) Supervision: a cooperative exercise in accountability. In: Marken, M., Payne, M. (eds.) *Enabling and Ensuring.* Leicester: Leicester National Youth Bureau and Council for Education and Training in Youth and Community Work.

Roper, N., Logan, W., Tierney, A. (1985) *The Elements of Nursing.* Edinburgh: Churchill Livingstone.

Roy, C. (1984) *Introduction to Nursing: An Adaptation Model.* Englewood Cliffs, NJ: Prentice Hall.

Schon, D. (1983) *The Reflective Practitioner.* New York, NY: Basic Books.

United Kingdom Central Council for Nursing, Midwifery and Health Visiting (1992) *Code of Professional Conduct.* London: UKCC.

United Kingdom Central Council for Nursing, Midwifery and Health Visiting (1996) *Position Statement on Clinical Supervision for Nursing and Health Visiting.* London: UKCC.

Wolsey, P., Leach, L. (1997) Clinical supervision: a hornet's nest? *Nursing Times*; 93, 44 .

4 Implementing supervision – cases and examples

Sarah Adams

This chapter offers some examples of the implementation of clinical supervision in a variety of practice areas and offers some suggestions for implementation. It is not intended to act as a template and those who wish to implement supervision in their workplace must make the model of supervision fit the workplace, not the other way round.

CLINICAL SUPERVISION AND THE PRACTICE NURSE

The extended or expanded role of the practice nurse has been of some concern to the nursing profession and the individual alike. With the introduction of *The Scope of Professional Practice* (UKCC, 1992) it became apparent that it would be more difficult for the practice nurse to say no to the general practitioner, who may request that the practice nurse perform tasks for which they are not adequately trained.

There are other reasons for the vulnerability of practice nurses, not least their lack of management structure, as they tend to be managed by their medical colleagues (Cook, 1992), and absence of support from their health authorities, some of whom have little recognised support for practice nurses. Practice nurses are not paid in a uniform way, an issue currently under discussion. In addition to this there is as yet no uniform scheme or educational initiative to ensure practice nurse competency when entering employment. Many practice nurses gain formal education from a variety of schemes, ranging from study days sponsored by pharmaceutical firms to modular university diplomas whose philosophy is often based on research-based practice in an environment of shared learning.

The role of the practice nurse

Unfortunately, the role of the practice nurse is not well defined; for many it is formed largely on the foundations of *Promoting Better Health* (Department of Health, 1987) which encouraged a new perspective with the promotion of health and prevention of disease. This involved screening, health promotion and immunisation initiatives. At this point it became clear that general practitioners would need further professional help to provide the service that was expected. Until recently, the role of the practice nurse was often moulded by practice budgets and remuneration schemes. It may, therefore, be noted that this is a group of professionals who would have a lot to gain from clinical supervision.

The practicalities of clinical supervision in general practice

Getting started is the most difficult stage. The key to good clinical supervision is careful planning. Many nurses are in primary care work in isolation and questions will spring to mind, such as: Who can I get to supervise me? Where will the supervision come from? How will I get the time? To consider some of the issues involved consider this scenario.

Sandra's story

Sandra came into practice nursing from a midwifery background two years ago. She initially worked at a busy four-doctor practice at which her duties were mainly women's healthcare and general health promotion.

Sandra was comfortable in this role and had support from her nursing colleagues. She has now joined a small isolated rural practice in which her role is much more varied and is to include a child immunisation programme. Although she has a broad theoretical knowledge, she has no previous experience of performing immunisations to this group. Her GP has offered to lend a hand but has little experience in this field himself.

Possible approach

The UKCC Code of Professional Conduct for Nursing, Midwifery and Health Visiting Professions clearly places the responsibility for standards of care with the qualified practitioner and, as such, Sandra needs an immunisation programme she understands and feels competent using. Due to the size of the practice, Sandra is the sole nurse and works in isolation.

Who could supervise Sandra?

In clinical supervision it is not necessary for the supervisor to be of the same discipline as the person supervised. In this instance it made geographical and practical sense for Sandra to approach someone who was employed in the area. However, there was a local practice nurse group who met monthly 10 miles away. Sandra inquired and found it would be possible to use this as a backup system for group supervision. It would be impractical, if not impossible, for Sandra to attend group supervision regularly due to the isolated nature of the surgery. After some inquiry Sandra was directed towards the health visitor who was based in the village. The clinical supervision was to take the form of mainly one-to-one supervision.

How could the supervision take place?

Much discussion was needed to deliberate this point as Sandra was employed by the general practitioner and the health visitor by the local health trust. As a result, both professionals had different demands and were accountable to different managers. It became evident that the baby clinic and the immunisation clinic would need to be combined in order that both professionals maximise their skills and time. A suitable time and location would be fixed. It was also agreed that both parties would have the support of the practice nurse forum group, many of whom were experienced in running immunisation programme. Using one or more supervisors is usually described as network supervision. This model enables the provision of particular areas of expertise or skills when needed in an individual way within the remit of clinical supervision. Practice nurses may link in an organised way across the district or locality (Cook, 1995).

How could the supervision evolve?

There are several opportunities for supervision in this situation. The provision of the clinic immediately fits the criteria for **live** supervision. This is an ongoing process and occurs simultaneously with practice being supervised. There may be an opportunity following the clinic for **immediate** supervision. This is the term used for a supervision session that takes place very soon after the practice on which it is to focus. **Delayed** supervision may be integrated into the supervision sessions with the nurse forum group. Here Sandra can bring past events to discuss with the supervising nurses. For such a visit at infrequent intervals Sandra may find a diary of events a beneficial aid when attempting to recall events or feelings.

Evaluation

Sandra needs clinical supervision for this particular role and has implemented it. However, it is important to remember that clinical practice should not only promote professionally accountable practitioners, but also sustain and develop practice. As Sandra is responsible for her own practice development it would seem natural to develop this situation to incorporate PREP (UKCC, 1990). Clinical audit may form a baseline from where clinical supervision can be measured and Sandra may find this a useful tool with which to improve or make amendments to the service currently offered.

CLINICAL SUPERVISION AND THE CRITICAL CARE NURSE

The critical care speciality is considered by many as being an area of high stress. As therapeutic techniques become ever more complex and new practices and technology advance, so critical care nurses must adapt to an ever-developing service. Critical care nurses often find themselves judged not by the care itself but by the outcome of that care, in an area already full of intense emotion caring for the most vulnerable and dependent of people. Critical care nurses must be prepared for their care and speciality as a whole to remain under scrutiny, not only from politicians but also from hospital managers and anxious relatives alike. Specialist skills in the detailed observation and management of patients need to be developed, including the utilisation of the technology available and the ever-necessary counselling skills. For an area such as this, clinical supervision is paramount.

The role of the critical care nurse

The role of the critical care nurse has evolved in response to changes in healthcare. There is a driving force towards clinical specialisation and in critical care we can clearly see that which used to be regarded as the extended clinical role being accepted as an integral part of daily patient care (Mechanic, 1988). Critical care nurses must set and demonstrate high standards of nursing care and strive to maintain these. There is an ever-increasing diversity of knowledge base and increased focus on providing emotional support for patients. However, some nurses in a critical care area may become preoccupied with technical competency to the detriment of humanistic caring.

The practicalities of clinical supervision in a critical care unit

Much of the role of the critical care nurse will be open to supervision. Due to the geographic layout in intensive care units often there may be opportunities for one-to-one supervision in 'live' situations. However, critical care nurses are frequently in need of support to develop the skills for holistic care, enabling nurses to develop the skills to meet the individual needs of patients.

Charles' story

Charles has worked as a critical care nurse for seven years and openly admits he likes the technology. Although it is a stressful area this has been something which, until recently, he has thrived on. Recently, Charles has found himself admitting that he is drawn to patients that require his technical abilities rather than his humanity. After attending a study day with other disciplines he came away feeling rather deflated as he had recognised some deterioration in his 'caring' skills. Charles is a senior nurse and is now attempting to address his problem.

Possible approach

In this situation Charles does not have to choose a supervisor for clinical knowledge of his chosen area. He has a need to relate how he feels about his role, and may need to address his caring skills. As a senior nurse he will have knowledge of internal and external agencies that may be of benefit to him. Charles has the experience and maturity to realise that he has a broad knowledge of clinical practice that brings much expertise to the critical care unit. He is mature enough to accept responsibility for maintaining his own practice and may seek supervision from a variety of sources.

Who could supervise Charles?

The whole environment of critical care depends on good teamwork; members in critical care work closely together to evaluate and plan patient care. As he is a more senior member of staff, Charles may prefer to share his concerns with a member less involved in the daily running and staff relationships. He may decide to approach a colleague of a similar grade from another discipline. Alternatively, Charles could utilise the role of the clinical nurse specialist (CNS). Clinical nurse specialists are nurses who 'demonstrate refined clinical practice as a result of significant experience, advanced expertise or knowledge of a particular branch or speciality' (Royal College of Nursing, 1988). The CNS must therefore be instrumental in the maintenance of high standards of care and practice in the critical care area. A CNS would recognise the importance of potential 'burn out' in such an area and the support necessary to prevent this.

How could the supervision take place?

The supervision would be on a one-to-one basis, as the CNS should practise on the unit. It would be possible for live supervision, with the two of them working together. However, if Charles finds this a little intimidating, a series of reflections on case studies could be arranged so that appropriate issues could be discussed. Alternatively, they may decide to follow one patient and evaluate their needs and plan the implementation of care as an ongoing supervision.

How could the supervision evolve?

The CNS has a broad understanding of all aspects of critical care and may be able to recognise problems that Charles has not yet addressed. For instance, Charles may be taking more than his share of the workload, which does not allow time for the patient care, or there may be ways of rearranging the staffing to allow the trained nurses more time for patient care. It may be necessary to address the situation in more depth and measure whether the rest of the trained staff also feel this way. The CNS could be used as a catalyst for opening such a discussion between staff.

Evaluation

By approaching the CNS, who has a slightly removed insight of critical care nursing, Charles not only enables himself to gain support and improve his caring skills, but also brings the topic to the attention of the person who values staff insights and may be able to address the problem on a broader scale.

CLINICAL SUPERVISION AND THE HEALTH VISITOR

The latest edition of the Hall Report (1996) reflects a shifting emphasis away from child health surveillance and screening towards a greater focus on primary prevention. The importance of evidence-based practice is stressed and the difficulties in measuring child health work are brought to the forefront.

Health visitors and other professionals alike are encouraged to give greater emphasis to the mental health of the child and to forge supportive partnerships with parents. The report also calls for all health service staff to collaborate with other agencies to provide a coordinated service promoting child health.

The role of the health visitor is ever evolving, with many health visitors now offering specialist advice in the home or in clinic settings. In some instances health visitors have developed these roles with theoretical knowledge and enthusiasm alone. As most health visitors are usually designated a caseload it is a profession used to a large degree of autonomy. As all health visitors are registered nurses they are aware of the need for clinical supervision. The child protection component of this supervision is usually the responsibility of the senior nurse or the team leader who is guided by the recommendations from the HMSO publication, *Guidance for Senior Nurses, Health Visitors and Midwives* (1996).

The role of the health visitor

The health visitor works within the primary health team to promote health, identify health needs and work with all clients to promote and safeguard their wellbeing and interests. This will empower the client to reach their optimum level of health through health education advice and promotion. The health visitor's remit appears huge for any one professional, thus it is paramount that the practitioner feels confident in their abilities to work within their own capabilities and to refer to other agencies if necessary. *The Scope of Professional Practice* (UKCC, 1992) states firm recommendations that must be met before adjusting the scope of practice, but then proceeds to make a special case for health visitors stating: 'There are frequent occasions when the full contributions of health visitors may not find expression where it is most needed... There is merit in allowing health visitors, where they judge it appropriate, to use their full range of skills in response to needs identified in pursuit of their health visiting practice.'

The practicalities of clinical supervision in the health visitor role

Many trusts have begun to instigate some form of clinical supervision in the community. Most health visitors work within a community team and have accessibility to peer review, but a functioning supportive team capable of providing high quality clinical supervision unfortunately is not always the reality for many health visitors who can at times feel alone and isolated with a difficult and concerning caseload.

Kate's story

Kate is a health visitor and also a team leader. As such she has a divided role between management and client-based work. Recently, Kate has been involved in a child protection case, which is now proceeding to a criminal court case in which Kate may be called to give evidence. Although Kate has worked in child protection many times, this case has become more protracted and complicated than any she has been involved in before. She is feeling under considerable pressure and really just needs a little moral support and guidance from someone with suitable knowledge.

Possible approach

Kate has already proved her competencies in this field but needs reassurance with this client workload. In particular she is concerned that her record keeping should be flawless and withstand scrutiny. She clearly has many avenues to take for clinical supervision with an extended community team and close links with other involved agencies.

Who could supervise Kate?

It has been suggested that there are disadvantages to management supervision (Butterworth et al, 1997) and that the management agenda may dominate to the detriment of the supervisee's agenda. In this situation, however, the senior nurse in this area is also designated as the clinical supervisor for child protection and, as such, has an abundance of knowledge and advice. The advantage of Kate choosing her manager in this instance is that she is aware of the contextual issues locally and may be useful in relation to accessing internal and external networks for the supervisee.

How could the supervision take place?

Due to the demands on the time of both these professionals it would seem justified to have a formal time prearranged and agreed by both parties. This may not necessarily need to be on a regular basis, as it may only be necessary as events unfold. It may be that determining a regular plan beforehand would enable anticipation of events surrounding the case that could be discussed during supervision. The manager who is supervisor must be prepared for the role and in this case the designated nurse for child protection should be trained in an advisory role.

How could the supervision evolve?

Proactive supervision may be appropriate in this situation. This supervision usually occurs in more advanced forms of supervision, but the fundamentals involve the supervisor recognising issues proactively. This allows for rehearsals of possible courses of action that may be effective if anticipated issues or events occur in the future. If the situation becomes very intense, this may then revert back to a form of live clinical supervision whereby the clinical nurse could actually involve herself in the fieldwork to actively support Kate.

Evaluation

Kate needed support for a stressful situation and in this instance was able to use management levels. Although guidance on a practical level may not have been her primary concern, by using clinical supervision Kate was able to benefit by broadening her thinking and increasing her commitment and professionalism. At the same time, she was able to promote her self-assurance and increase her confidence. As a result she was able to continue to enhance patient care and continue her involvement with the family.

CLINICAL SUPERVISION IN THE OUTPATIENTS DEPARTMENT

Outpatients departments are, for many members of the public, the first experience and contact with the local hospital on a personal level. The clients have often waited for long periods just to reach the outpatients department before they are given any further explanation or treatment. They may be anxious and disillusioned with the healthcare available. Clinic staff are under ever-increasing pressure to allocate appropriate appointments so that waiting lists and care in the clinic are realistically comparable with the descriptions in the hospital or health authority patients' charter. The general public are becoming ever more aware of their rights, and justifiably so. However, patient empowerment is often not compatible with lack of clinic appointments or staff in the clinic. Clinic nurses are in the front line for dealing with political and often very emotive issues.

The role of the outpatient department nurse

Many outpatient departments now increasingly rely on unqualified staff, with the numbers of trained staff declining in most cases. The advantages and disadvantages of this can be argued, but the fact remains that qualified nurses are functioning more and more in an administrative and managerial role, responsible for the overall running of the clinic. They are now responsible for the development of staff, standard setting, policies and procedures and clinical audit. These processes help both to evaluate the care provided for the patients and to supply the benchmarks for quality assurance programmes. Such programmes are becoming a fundamental part of healthcare today and in 1996 the UKCC stated: Nurses should be 'aware of the current policy debates that shape their work. They will need tools to evaluate their own practice and the skills to argue the case for a particular service and to defend it against criticism' (UKCC, 1996). For outpatient nurses the evaluation of services has become a very topical issue.

The practicalities of clinical supervision in an outpatient department

Practical supervision is not always easy in this environment. Often the clinic nurse works alone and may not have access to a supervisor for live supervision. Many clinic nurses rely on managers for guidance and for a large part of their role development.

Julia's story

Julia is an experienced staff nurse who has practised in orthopaedics for three years and has recently moved to the outpatients' area. She is mainly involved with the orthopaedic and trauma clinics and on the whole has no problems; she regards herself as a competent clinic nurse. However, after a few months Julia becomes increasingly aware that the information given to the patients in clinic regarding their impending treatment is often scanty, and on occasion wholly incorrect. Julia finds this very frustrating as patients often complain about conflicting information. Julia believes this causes antagonism and frustration not only in the clinic, but also on the orthopaedic wards. The information is relayed by a number of different sources. Julia feels she needs some guidance to find a solution to this.

Possible approach

Before Julia can address the problem of finding a clinical supervisor she needs to determine what the problem actually is. Is this really a problem or has she perceived it to be a problem? For the answer to this question she could undertake a clinical audit to clarify the situation. By using this method she would become more aware of the issues involved and where she could find the best supervision.

Who could supervise Julia?

Julia could possibly use a manager or another member of staff from the clinic for her clinical supervision. However, as the issue stands at present it would seem logical to address the problem systematically. She may gain great insight from studying other outpatient services in the hospital and having discussions with staff in these areas to determine how to manage the communication issues. Added to this, Julia may decide to inquire on a broader basis to find a suitable programme or technique, and then search for the available support to implement it.

How could the supervision take place?

Julia can approach other clinics in her hospital and make arrangements to visit or to request information from other units. There will have been much research in the area of communication and patient satisfaction. Julia would be able to gain support from a nurse tutor or an experienced colleague on the best way to approach this topic. Network supervision (accepting supervision from outside sources) works by providing the occasional input of an outside view.

How could the supervision evolve?

As Julia becomes more aware of the issues involved she will gain confidence in approaching a supervisor. By using outside influences she can view the problem objectively, and will have the benefit of other working models. If the audit identifies a need, Julia can then seek support for implementation of the necessary policies and protocols. During the course of this external supervision she can use group discussion with her work colleagues as a form of immediate supervision of the audit.

Evaluation

Having identified a problem Julia approaches it in a professional manner. She incorporates the very fundamentals of clinical supervision by bringing practitioners and supervisors together to reflect on practice, to improve practice and to increase their understanding of professional issues.

CLINICAL SUPERVISION AND THE PSYCHIATRIC NURSE

The role of the psychiatric nurse has been affected by recent changes in the organisation of psychiatric services. The supervision register and supervised discharge have probably been one of the most controversial issues for psychiatric nurses in recent years. Mental health workers have used clinical supervision in one form or another for a number of years and there are many studies which argue the merits of formalised/non-formalised clinical supervision (Rushton, 1988) and the decision on whether to follow set models in doing so. There is also much literature describing the implications of clinical supervision and mental health nurses' perceptions of it (Scanlon and Weir, 1997). However, many of the problems that have afflicted the nursing profession as a whole, such as the very fact that we have gone from a position of apparently little interest to a veritable explosion of ideas, have left mental health nurses with the same headaches of implementation. Due to the very nature of the psychiatric nurse role, clinical supervision implemented badly may be not only constricting for the practitioner but also detrimental to the care of the patient.

The role of the psychiatric nurse

The role of the psychiatric nurse is split into three major sections: that related to **custodial care**, that which is supportive to a **medical model** and, perhaps most importantly, that which requires psychiatric nurses to **personally influence the mental health** of the patient. Possibly the primary function of the psychiatric nurse is a psychotherapeutic one, which has been described by various nursing theorists as relationship therapy, counselling and psychotherapy, and interpersonal relationships. Psychotherapy is often used to diagnose and influence patients' responses and perceptions of their mental health. The focus for the psychiatric nurse frequently arises from the concerns of clients, often observed using expertise in a client/practitioner interaction. Therapeutic skills, however, may be among the most difficult to evaluate, making it essential for the supervisor to have a reasonable understanding of the clinical role, and many theorists would argue that for psychiatry the teacher may fit the purpose of clinical supervisor.

The practicalities of clinical supervision for the psychiatric nurse

Many psychiatric nurses and nursing students are familiar with the concept of clinical supervision. Often these concepts are underpinned with nursing models or a multiplicity of theories. In 1988, Peplau suggested that the 'phenomena commonly observed by nurses in their relationships with psychiatric clients should be the focus for nursing intervention and the clinical supervision of learners'. In real terms this is costly, advocating one-to-one supervision. Many psychiatric nurses complain the situation is one of too few knowledgeable and skilled nurses to supervise those in need.

Brett's story

Brett is a newly qualified psychiatric nurse. He is currently employed on a busy admissions ward. As he is employed at the hospital he trained in he is well aware of the formal clinical supervision process, but he feels that it is not implemented in real terms. There is a chronic shortage of trained nurses and many of the experienced staff lack skills in supervision, as they sometimes confuse the issue with management proceedings and disciplinary measures. Brett finds himself asking his peers that qualified at the same time as him for advice and support. Often it is purely reassurance of case management that he requires, and he feels frustrated that this is not readily available.

Possible approach

Brett needs an opportunity to discuss individual client cases; he is disillusioned with the clinical supervision structure. He needs to seek supervision from an alternative source, but with a shortage of trained nurses this may prove difficult.

Who could supervise Brett?

The majority of nursing theorists and teachers of psychiatric nursing agree that it is beneficial for the teacher or supervisor to be working in the clinical environment. As Brett is newly qualified his supervision needs will change as he increases his experience and gains confidence. Other peer members who qualified at the same time will possibly be experiencing the same problems. Although somewhat lacking in experience, these peers will have a wealth of knowledge which can be pooled in an effective way. Brett could gain his support from a group forum (made up from peers) that could discuss individual case studies or focus on a particular phenomenon experienced.

How could the supervision take place?

Group forums can meet at set times to suit the group members. This method of supervision surmounts some of the issues surrounding time commitment and the number of supervisors required. This group would come together specifically for the purposes of clinical supervision.

How could the supervision evolve?

Issues and experiences are shared in a group forum. It should be acknowledged that some of the issues it seeks to address might not be easily raised in this type of supervision. However, by limiting this group to peers the group becomes less intimidating. As the group grows in confidence they may choose to invite an external facilitator or supervisor, but it should be remembered that this person needs not only the skills for supervision but also for group facilitation.

Evaluation

Brett now has the benefit of a formal clinical supervisor in the less formal environment of the group forum. When embarking on such a project ambitious plans should be rejected and the group should concentrate on the needs of its members. As the newly qualified nurses' confidence grows they may feel the need for such a group decreases; indeed the group may come to a natural end.

CONCLUSION

As mentioned above, the situations offered as thought provoking scenarios are just that. It must be remembered that for supervision to work you need to create a system that:

▶ meets the needs of the staff;

▶ can be achieved within the workplace environment;

▶ has clear benefits for the client group.

Be as flexible and creative as possible in the ways you try to implement supervision. Do not be afraid to take chances with supervision and do not hesitate to change and adapt the way that supervision is used where you work. Above all, give it a try. You will not be disappointed with what you can achieve.

REFERENCES

Butterworth, T., Carson, J., White, E. et al (1997) *It's Good to Talk: Clinical Supervision and Mentorship. An Evaluation Study in England and Scotland.* Manchester: University of Manchester.

Cook, R. (1992) Healthy new arrivals. *Practice Nurse*; 3: 7, 12–15.

Cook, R. (1995) Clinical supervision and practice nurses. *Practice Nurse*; 6: 2, 31–34.

Department of Health (1987) *Promoting Better Health.* London: HMSO.

Hall, M.B. (1996) *Health For All Children.* (3rd edition) Oxford: Oxford University Press.

HMSO (1996) *Guidance for Senior Nurses, Health Visitors and Midwives.* London: HMSO.

Mechanic, H. (1988) Redefining the expanded role. *Nursing Outlook*; 36, 280–284.

NHS Executive (1997) *Clinical Supervision: A Resource Pack for Practice Nurses.* London: NHS Executive.

Peplau, H. (1988) *Substance and Scope of Psychiatric Nursing.* Paper presented at the Third Conference of Psychiatric Nursing. Montreal.

Royal College of Nursing (1988) *Specialities of Nursing.* London: RCN.

Rushton, B. (1988) Implementing a reflective model of care within a community mental health team. *Mental Health Care*; 1: 9, 300–302.

Scanlon, C., Weir, W.S. (1997) Learning from practice? Mental health nurses' perceptions and experiences of clinical supervision. *Journal of Advanced Nursing*; 26: 2, 295–303.

United Kingdom Central Council for Nursing, Midwifery and Health Visiting (1990) *The Report of the Post Registration Education Practice Project.* London: UKCC.

United Kingdom Central Council for Nursing, Midwifery and Health Visiting (1992) *The Scope of Professional Practice.* London: UKCC.

United Kingdom Central Council for Nursing, Midwifery and Health Visiting (1996) *Guidelines for Professional Practice.* London: UKCC.

5 Barriers to clinical supervision

Mac Macintosh and Mick Ashman

In recent years there has been a great deal of literature giving advice on the process of change – so much so that the thought of reading yet another chapter on this subject will probably not elicit much enthusiasm. The objective is not, therefore, to indulge in a further descriptive account of the change process but rather to concentrate on exploring some of the reasons why this particular change, at this time and in this profession, may come up against barriers. Any discussion of barriers, by the very nature of the topic, runs the risk of seeming pessimistic and negative. This is not the intention here; our aim is to provide an illustration of the type of analysis one must undertake if one is seriously attempting to introduce a complex innovation. While the precise nature of the barriers faced will inevitably be determined by the type of area into which the development is being introduced, there are likely to be a number of themes that are common across many areas. Identification and analysis of potential barriers is always a key part of the implementation process.

MODELS OF CHANGE

Lewin's (1951) classic model of change proposes that for change to take place 'driving forces', that is the forces that are supporting the change, must overcome the resistance, or barriers, to the change. It has been suggested that the dominant approach to overcoming resistance, or barriers, is to increase the driving forces to a point where they overwhelm the resistance (Pryjmachuk, 1996). Perhaps a better approach is to try to dismantle the barriers (Argyris, 1970); indeed, such a strategy fits more closely with the philosophy that underpins clinical supervision. The first step then is to identify the potential barriers to the change. Once identified an analysis of the reasons why such barriers exist allows strategies to be developed that may be used to remove them.

CLINICAL SUPERVISION AND CHANGE

Clinical supervision is new in the field of nursing. It could be looked on as an innovation and as such may suffer from some of the problems of any 'new idea'. Introducing something new means change, and here lies the problem.

It seems that 'change' has developed a reputation for being problematic. Most writers on change and change theory talk of change being treated with suspicion, of causing uncertainty and even fear, to the point where one comes away from the literature with the impression that any change will be viewed as something negative until proven otherwise (for example, Wright, 1998). Why is this? Why should the concept of change, even change that has the potential to improve our situation, have come to have developed such a negative image when applied to the organisations in which we work?

The answer is complex and needs to be examined from both a general and a specific viewpoint. What is it about change in general that makes it difficult, what is it about change in nursing, and what is it about a change to clinical supervision that may cause problems in implementation?

The problems of change

Modern organisations are today expected to embrace change as a constant part of their development and this reflects much of modern life (Handy, 1993; Peters, 1988; Kanter, 1983). We are exposed constantly to change at a pace that is almost too fast to deal with. Technology, employment, leisure and so on, all seem to be in a constant state of change. It feels that as soon as we have come to terms with, for example, a new information management system at work, it changes and there is a new system to learn. This appears to be going on around us, with us in the middle trying to keep up. Such a sensation is uncomfortable at the very least, fearful at worst. Why should this be uncomfortable?

Control

A simple response is to consider change in relation to control. Of how many of the major changes in your work over the past 10 years have you felt in control? Is it not a common criticism that many of the changes that affect our lives, our working lives in particular, are imposed rather than voluntarily embraced? Psychologists have shown that we view lack of control as a threat, that it creates feelings that are negative, and that our natural instincts will be to avoid it (Lazerus and Lannier, 1981). When the threat is a change that is being introduced that we feel little control over, it creates key problems. The feelings of threat that are generated are unpleasant and we tend to associate these feelings with the thing that is causing the threat, that is the change. From the point of view of those responsible for introducing the change, in this case clinical supervision, once such feelings and associations are generated you are faced with a mountain to climb. Stop for a moment and imagine your reaction to someone trying to get you to be supportive and enthusiastic about something that makes you feel threatened and uncomfortable. This issue of control is fundamental to the successful implementation of any change, particularly something that has the characteristics of clinical supervision, as we shall see later. So the first principle would seem to be to avoid creating such feelings to begin with. This is not easy, as there will undoubtedly be a certain amount of prejudging.

Costs and benefits

A second important principle is that change inevitably has costs. The benefits of the change have to be seen to be worth the costs. The costs incurred in change are complex and are not just financial. There are costs in terms of time and effort, and in indirect resources. There may also be psychological costs in terms of the feelings of uncertainty that can be generated. There may even be a sense of loss; to embrace something new often means leaving something old behind – 'What was wrong with how things used to be?' Such feelings of nostalgia are common when faced with a complicated and uncertain future.

For the individual faced with the transition that is inevitably a part of coping with change there will be, some have suggested, a cycle of reactions that is predictable (Adams et al, 1976). Adams et al describe a number of stages that are moved through when faced with changes that are related to self-esteem. The first of these is 'immobilisation' or shock, the characteristics of which are an inability to plan and to reason, followed by a stage of minimisation, where the impact is denied or ignored. Following this minimisation stage there is a stage of depression, and with this stage comes a lowering of self-esteem as it is realised that one may have no control over events and the reality of the transition becomes apparent. Eventually self-esteem is restored as the change becomes accepted and incorporated into one's behaviour. The depth of these feelings, and the speed with which the transition evolves, will be affected by the degree of familiarity with, and the expectations of, the change; the more unfamiliar and the more negative the expectations the deeper the sense of immobilisation, denial and subsequent depression. Those involved in implementing change need to be aware of the very real psychological threat that change may trigger.

A change such as clinical supervision is entirely dependent for its success on it having the support of the people using it. The attitude to the change must be a positive one for it to have a realistic chance of working. This positive attitude cannot be taken for granted. The costs incurred are real to people and the benefits are not always easy to see straight away. It is essential though that a positive attitude to the change is generated from the start.

This will be influenced largely by the way the change is presented to and perceived by those who are to be affected. An oversimplified but useful approach is to ask yourself: 'Is this going to be seen as a threat or an opportunity?' In his influential book *Future Shock*, Toffler (1973) suggested that both in and out of work we have what have been described as 'safety zones': those places, people, procedures and practices that are familiar and therefore comfortable and 'safe'. When we come to implement clinical supervision we are probably asking people to step out of a 'safety zone' and to embark on something new and unfamiliar. Whether they do so willingly and with enthusiasm will be the determining factor in successful implementation. People will largely view what is on offer outside their safety zone as either threat or opportunity. This threat or opportunity is then weighed against the costs. Later we will be looking at ways of creating a sense of opportunity rather than threat, and of minimising the costs and maximising the perception of benefit.

▶ Change can be threatening.

▶ Change has costs.

▶ Change may make people feel out of control.

▶ Change may feel like loss.

▶ When faced with uncertainty people tend to retreat to their 'safety zones'.

We next need to consider the cultural environment into which we are to introduce the change of clinical supervision – the climate of nursing and healthcare. Much has been written about the problems encountered when implementing change in nursing, so much so that one comes away with quite a negative image (for example, Walsh and Ford, 1989). Is this perception fair and, if so, why is it like this? We will see that there are clear historical reasons and it is important to consider the ways in which our past may continue to present us with potential barriers to change.

NURSING AS A CHANGE CULTURE

Bureaucracy

Modern organisations need to develop cultures where change is the norm, where innovation occurs naturally and painlessly, if they are to survive and develop (Handy, 1993). This is truer now than ever, and nursing and health must respond to this challenge.

What sort of cultural background is nursing emerging from that may impact on its ability to accept change in a positive way?

Nursing has developed within the framework of the National Health Service (NHS) and NHS hospitals. Both the NHS and hospitals have been identified as having many of the characteristics of bureaucracy (Lawton and Rose, 1991). The term 'bureaucracy' tends to be used pejoratively but describes a type of organisational structure with characteristics of hierarchy, discipline, rigid rules and regulations, impersonality of managers and fixed and limited official duties (Beetham, 1989). Many of our large organisations were built on such principles and many still retain at least some of these characteristics despite recent moves to flatten our structures and embrace modern organisational principles. Nursing has its modern roots in such organisations, which in part accounts for the view of nursing as having been a very hierarchical, rule-based profession (Salvage, 1984). Change and innovation in such cultures tends to be top-down and imposed using power-coercive strategies; bottom-up innovative change tends to be less likely. Modern organisational theories tell us that innovation will occur, and the workforce will respond positively to change and development, in organisations based on participation and devolved management and decision-making (Kanter, 1983).

Subordination

Apart from the organisational structures and culture there are other compounding reasons why nursing has been a fairly traditional, slow changing and subordinate profession. Two of the most influential are our historical subordination to medicine (Hegman, 1994), and having a predominantly female workforce with all the societal norms of undervaluing of what is seen as 'women's work' (Jones, 1994; Salvage, 1984). We have suffered from both the tendency to allow medicine to control decision-making and the perception that, while society may value nursing and nurses, it is in a manner which is affectionate rather than as a credible, high status profession. A workforce that is continually looking to others to guide and control it, and which sees itself as a rather passive, if well-loved, workhorse was unlikely to have the self-confidence to foster innovation and a positive, proactive approach to change. The question that asks, 'How far have we moved from this position?' is not easily answered.

The combination of a rule-based hierarchy and traditional subordination may have had the effect of creating a number of key problems that acted as barriers to change. Importantly, the management style that arises from such circumstances is often one that is based on control and discipline. Research has demonstrated that in such a climate change is more likely to be treated with suspicion when suggested from above, and unlikely to emerge from below. This is perhaps because it is seen as risk taking or 'sticking your neck out' (see 'Tall Poppy Syndrome', Faugier, 1993) and because creativity and initiative tend to be stifled. While the profession has undoubtedly moved on from this position, one must be aware that vestiges of this culture will still remain and that cultural change in large organisations is invariably slow. It is still only quite recently that Walsh and Ford (1989) exposed the reality of the traditional and reactionary culture that pervaded nursing and was creating a very real barrier to change.

Size and diversity

The size and diversity of the nursing profession may also have contributed to a work culture that has a tendency to treat change with suspicion. As the profession has grown it has inevitably fragmented and developed a range of separate identities. Mental health nursing, health visiting, accident and emergency nursing, operating department nursing and occupational health nursing all have their own particular identity and culture within the broader framework of nursing. While this is necessary and desirable to a point, it has introduced an element of competitiveness and insecurity that may add to any sense of mistrust of change that already exists. The different areas of specialism within nursing are vying with each other for resources, credibility and recognition. As each new area of specialism emerges it quickly establishes its own associations, conferences and study days, perhaps motivated in part by a need to demonstrate to itself and to others the uniqueness of its particular area. When faced with a profession-wide innovation each separate group will need to reassure itself that this is right for them, that this is not something that other groups have developed that may not fit with their particular needs. We have seen examples of this potential barrier in the tension that exists between nursing and midwifery. An innovation emerging from a nursing development might not be appropriate with a midwifery setting, and vice versa. The potential is that *all* innovations emerging from a part of nursing different to one's own are viewed with suspicion. Such a position would undoubtedly be seen as a barrier to successful implementation. Kanter (1983) has identified a similar culture occurring within many organisations that she has called 'segmentalism': the notion that problems and developments are seen too narrowly, are only seen within the context of one's own particular 'segment' of the organisation. The alternative culture is one of integration, what Kanter calls 'integrative' cultures. In such cultures innovation and change are seen in a holistic way, with benefits and barriers for the whole organisation, as opposed to just one's own part of it, being considered.

Research culture

The move to a research-based culture is quite new and many, if not most, nurses have neither trained nor worked within a culture of research-based evidence until recently. By examining our recent history we can see that the notion of providing convincing reliable evidence to support our innovations is relatively new. In the past we were prepared neither to provide the evidence nor to ask for it. This has changed but our past still resonates through many within the profession who feel threatened by, or at least uncomfortable with, the language of research (Carter, 1996). This may have now led to the situation where the person who does try to implement change, by presenting appropriate evidence, may be faced with resistance. Paradoxically, what is expected of a new idea is that it is scrutinised for evidence of its value and effectiveness before staff are expected to adopt it. On the one hand we are trying to bring a level of analysis to our innovations that was previously missing, and yet on the other we are trying not to alienate those who are still unfamiliar with the notion of providing appropriate evidence.

While the above discussion may appear to view the profession negatively, we have to recognise that despite the considerable steps forward nursing has made, it would be naive to assume that the developments of the past few years have had the same impact throughout the profession. The cultural background of the past is still with us and will continue to create barriers for some time.

- Nursing's hierarchical past may still influence how we view change.
- Our organisations have only recently begun to embrace ideas of participation.
- We have a history of leaving decision-making to our medical colleagues.
- Nursing's traditional history is not one of self-confidence.
- Tensions between specialisms may lead to suspicion.
- We may still be wary of people presenting research-based innovation.

Having acknowledged that the past has created problems for nursing and its ability to generate change we need to recognise that the NHS and nursing have experienced significant developments over the last 10 years and will continue to do so.

CHANGES IN ORGANISATIONAL STRUCTURE

The NHS has experienced significant organisational change over the last 10 years. The creation of the first NHS trusts in 1991, with the new emphasis on formal contracting arrangements between purchasers (health authorities) and providers (trusts), has been one of the factors contributing to examination by senior hospital managers of service configuration. The reforms placed a requirement on trusts to involve senior medical staff in service management; a move that led to creation of directorates and clinical management teams in most trusts. This reconfiguration resulted in a degree of 'flattening' of the traditional bureaucratic structure and allowed directorates to make some of their decisions independent of formal trust board approval. In some trusts such reconfiguration led to some managerial responsibilities being passed on to more junior staff; a move that was sometimes opposed by staff and their representative organisations (Cunningham, 1993). However, literature dealing with organisational structure supports the view that change is more likely to occur where responsibility and decision-making are devolved in this way (Handy, 1993).

Whether this 'flatter', less bureaucratic configuration has actually made change and development more likely is questionable. Anecdotal evidence suggests that although downward devolution of responsibility has created freedom from what were previous organisational constraints this has lead to an increased burden at ward level. Furthermore, according to a recent study by Marsh et al (in press), while the single highest ranked barrier to the implementation of new research-based ideas was insufficient time, when organisational constraints (such as lack of management support and leadership, and lack of support from medical colleagues) were grouped collectively these constituted the greatest barrier. The study would seem to support the view that despite organisational reconfiguration, wards and directorates themselves have tended to retain characteristics of the bureaucratic culture described earlier, and to retain a strong medical dominance. An interesting and related issue has been identified by Dunn et al (1997) and Walsh (1997), in that one of the main perceived barriers to the implementation of new practice was the fact that respondents did not feel that they had enough *authority* to change patient care procedures. Perhaps it is the case that despite developments in care delivery, in the organisation of nursing and the equal role of nursing within the multidisciplinary team, nurses continue to exhibit a lack of belief in their ability to affect change.

Managerialism

Paradoxically, the NHS reforms of the past two decades may have provided their own barriers. There has been a well-documented growth of a culture of management within the health service, stemming initially from the general management principles of the Griffith Report (DHSS, 1983), and developing within a model of what has been called 'new public management' (Hood, 1991). Those in management positions have had to operationalise the principles of the quasi-market, with its emphasis on output and results, competition and fiscal discipline, and some have argued that this has been achieved through the adoption of 'hard line managerialism' (Timpson, 1996). Whether or not one fully accepts this analysis, it is probably true that NHS management has come to be perceived as being overly preoccupied with cost and quantitatively based performance. This is combined with a feeling of management being distant from the realities of clinical practice (Cunningham, 1993), perhaps in part created by the increase in the use of the 'language' of management, and with the perception of many that those managing nursing either do not have, or have left behind, any clinical background. These factors have led to a situation where there seems to be an uncomfortable tension within the management of nursing. Recent studies have shown that there is a significant number of nurses who feel that those in management positions are not approachable, do not communicate well with the workforce and are less than supportive (Williams et al, 1998). In such a climate any change that is seen as being top-down may be viewed with suspicion simply because it is coming from 'above', that is coming from management (Nolan et al, 1998). If clinical supervision is perceived by staff as being imposed in such a way, it will invariably meet with resistance.

Morale

It is probably obvious that a workforce that is suffering from problems of low morale will be unlikely to be enthusiastic about change, particularly when the change will involve extra work, time and resources. Unfortunately, it would appear that health service staff, in particular nurses, are struggling with a significant morale problem; a problem that is evident from recent studies of staff health and workplace satisfaction (Williams et al, 1998) and from the well-publicised recruitment and retention problems (Watson, 1998; News, 1998). The reasons for this are complex and, while outside the scope of this discussion, must be considered as a considerable barrier to the implementation of any change. The individual charged with the responsibility of seeking to implement clinical supervision will need to acknowledge this.

This may well be compounded by the additional problem that a recruitment crisis brings. Many areas are reporting significant shortfalls in recruitment, which will inevitably lead to staff shortages (Watson, 1998). When facing a period of chronic understaffing any attempt to introduce a major new strategy, particularly one that requires the investment of time in order to be effective, is unlikely to even be considered by a pressurised workforce.

Too much change

A final barrier to change, repeatedly cited, stems from the amount of change, both perceived and real, that has occurred in the health service in recent years. Hogan (1997) goes as far as to suggest that the creation of the internal market and the resulting developments constituted almost as much change to healthcare delivery as did the creation of the NHS in 1948. Many health service staff feel that they have been overwhelmed with change in recent years: change in the form of organisational structure, management culture, education and research; changes in roles and role responsibilities, and in career expectations and choices. The reality is, of course, that this is not about to stop; that, in fact, this is now the norm. The implementation of clinical supervision is just one of many changes and innovations that are competing for the finite energies and enthusiasm of a health service staff that is becoming increasingly burdened by expectations.

The latest NHS changes, arising from the white paper, *The New NHS: Modern, Dependable* (Department of Health, 1998), will place considerable demands on staff. While there is every reason to view these changes positively, and despite the support for clinical supervision that is enshrined within the philosophy of the new strategies, many nurses will see it as yet another government initiative that nurses have to implement.

The irony is that clinical supervision, if successfully implemented, could provide staff with the support needed to cope with the pressures of continuous change.

▶ While organisational structures have developed, there is evidence that staff confidence in change implementation remains low.

▶ The managerial culture that has developed in the past 20 years has brought a suspicion of management initiatives.

▶ The nursing profession is going through problems of low morale, compounded by difficulties in recruitment and retention.

▶ The NHS and nursing have been overwhelmed by change in recent years.

CLINICAL SUPERVISION

The Department of Health (1993) defines clinical supervision as 'a formal process of professional support and learning which enables individual practitioners to develop knowledge and competence, assume responsibility for their own practice and enhance consumer protection'. This notion, that clinical supervision has the potential to facilitate developments in practice, would suggest that its very implementation could help to contribute to the development of a culture where innovation is more likely.

Let us now consider whether there are any characteristics of clinical supervision that might create problems with its implementation.

There has been a significant increase in the amount of literature dealing with clinical supervision since the publication of *A Vision for the Future* (Department of Health, 1993). Most of these articles regard clinical supervision as a mechanism for providing formalised support between two or more professionals through the process of reflective practice. However, what they also reveal is a lack of consensus as to what clinical supervision involves in precise terms. This is probably because no single approach to clinical supervision is deemed to be universally suitable to all disciplines of nursing and health visiting. This lack of clarity gives rise to two significant problems. First, that nurses may be uncomfortable with the lack of explicit guidance and still be in the position of asking, 'But what is it?'. Second, what might be implemented in the name of clinical supervision could result in models being implemented that are not necessarily congruent with the underpinning philosophy.

The lack of a prescribed model also makes an assessment of the resource implications of clinical supervision difficult. Questions such as, 'How much time is involved?', 'How much documentation is there to complete?' and 'How frequently should meetings be held?' cannot be answered precisely. Indeed the notion that something might be introduced that will be hard to quantify in terms of its impact on costs is likely to give rise to anxieties regarding its implementation. As discussed earlier, part of accepting change involves a cost/benefit analysis; if the costs cannot be identified then this analysis will be based on only partial information. This is partly compounded by the lack of research evidence that is currently available to demonstrate the benefits of clinical supervision in contexts other than psychotherapy.

A key problem for clinical supervision lies with the use of the word 'supervision' and the fact that it has associations with managerial supervision (Wright et al, 1997). In a profession that has strong hierarchical overtones the notion of some 'additional form of supervision' is likely to be met with apprehension and even resistance. The UKCC recognised this and sought to address these and other such concerns in the *Position Statement on Clinical Supervision for Nursing and Health Visiting* (UKCC, 1996). This provided a clear statement to the effect that clinical supervision should not be seen as a formal appraisal system or a tool for the managerial control of staff. Nevertheless, as the tendency to introduce clinical supervision with supervisors holding senior grades to supervisees is commonplace, the potential for this to be seen as a management tool must be acknowledged.

Concerns surrounding the issue of confidentiality may create another barrier that will need to be addressed sensitively if it is to be overcome. Clinical supervision is seen by the UKCC as a means of fulfilling organisational (NHS) objectives by providing a 'skilled, aware and articulate workforce'; an outcome that is achieved because it provides a mechanism for staff support and development. In order for this process to take place effectively it requires staff to discuss openly all aspects of the knowledge, skills and attitudes that constitute practice. This openness has been encouraged in working models of clinical supervision through the setting of ground rules that include clear statements regarding the maintenance of confidentiality by both parties. There is, however, an assumption that nurses will be happy to discuss all aspects of care delivery, which may involve disclosing material that could put their clinical practice and credibility in doubt. If clinical supervision is to facilitate real staff development, then clearly it will require considerable trust on the part of both parties. Supervision arrangements are likely to be problematic where the need to maintain confidentiality is faced with issues regarding patient safety and in situations where bad practice has been disclosed. Furthermore, there might be circumstances when serious misconduct is disclosed during a clinical supervision interview.

A related issue that may also be considered a potential barrier is in the skills required by those who are to be supervisors. Taking on the role of a clinical supervisor will undoubtedly raise considerable anxieties in relation to expectations. Finding oneself in the situation of supervising others when one feels that one does not have the appropriate skills or knowledge would be daunting. These skills may be perceived as ranging from counselling skills to advisory skills to facilitative skills and it cannot be taken for granted that such skills are present in the potential supervisors, either individually or in groups. Some lessons can be drawn here from the implementation of staff appraisal systems where people found themselves undertaking appraisals when they had not been adequately prepared (McGee, 1993).

▶ There is a lack of clarity in relation to what clinical supervision is and what it is not.

▶ Clinical supervision may be seen as a management tool.

▶ There are important concerns about confidentiality and accountability.

▶ There are concerns about the knowledge and skills required by supervisors.

▶ The resource implications are not clear.

Clinical supervision presents a considerable, but not insurmountable, challenge. It is a complex innovation because there is no precise 'off the shelf' model that can be universally implemented, because the costs and benefits are largely unknown and because it is dependent on the skill and confidence of the workforce – skill that may not initially be there, and confidence that recent studies suggest is struggling. It seeks to explore nursing practice in a way that will only work in a climate of openness and trust; this climate too cannot be taken for granted.

One could take the view that the above analysis is either a realistic one or is overly pessimistic. Regardless of where one stands on this question, it is undoubtedly the case that at least some of the barriers discussed here are very real for many health service staff. Our profession is a complex one that carries with it a considerable history and which is currently experiencing the difficulties associated with widespread and repeated change. Trying to implement an innovation of the magnitude of clinical supervision is a considerable undertaking and one that requires careful planning. The first stage in this planning should be analysis of the potential problems that may act as barriers to success; these barriers are complex and need to be acknowledged and respected. The most recent health service developments (Department of Health, 1998) are underpinned by philosophies that are, in theory, supportive of the sort of climate where change is viewed positively and is considered the norm. Such a climate will not be created overnight, however, which leaves us having to implement clinical supervision during a period of considerable transition. This may prove to be one of the key hurdles in implementation. However, with the necessary resources, development and support clinical supervision may well be seen as a considerable opportunity by those with the vision to see past the barriers.

REFERENCES

Adams, J., Hayes, B., Hopson, B. (1976) *Transition: Understanding and Managing Personal Change*. London: Martin Robertson.

Argyris, C. (1970) *Intervention Theory and Method*. Reading: Addison-Wesley.

Beetham, D. (1989) *Bureaucracy*. Milton Keynes: Open University Press.

Carter, D. (1996) Barriers to the implementation of research findings in practice. *Nurse Researcher*; 4: 2, 30–40.

Cunningham, G. (1993) Management control systems in the NHS. *Nursing Standard*; 3, 35–37.

Department of Health (1989) *Working for Patients, Cmnd 555*. London: HMSO.

Department of Health (1993) *A Vision for the Future*. London: HMSO.

Department of Health (1998) *The New NHS: Modern, Dependable*. London: HMSO.

DHSS (1983) *NHS Management Inquiry Report DHSS DA 83; 38*. Chair Roy Griffiths. London: HMSO.

Dunn, V., Crichton, N., Roe, B. et al (1997) Using research for practice: a UK experience of the Barriers Scale. *Journal of Advanced Nursing*; 26: 6, 1203–1210.

Faugier, J. (1993) Tall Poppies. *Nursing Times*; 88: 50, 20.

Handy, C. (1989) *The Age of Unreason*. London: Business Books.

Handy, C. (1993) *Understanding Organisations*. (4th edition) London: Penguin Business.

Hegman, J. (1994) *Power in the Caring Professions*. New York, NY: John Wiley and Sons.

Hogan, K. (1997) Change in the NHS: strategies and prospects. In: Clerk, J., Copcutt, L. (eds.) *Management for Nurses and Health Care Professionals*. Edinburgh: Churchill Livingstone.

Hood, C. (1991) A public management for all seasons? *Public Administration*; 69, 3–19.

Jones, L.J. (1994) *The Social Context of Health and Health Work*. London: Macmillan.

Kanter, R.M. (1983) *The Change Masters: Corporate Entrepreneurs at Work*. London: Allen and Unwin.

Lawton, A., Rose, A. (1991) *Organisation and Management in the Public Sector*. London: Pitman.

Lazerus, R.S., Lannier, R. (1981) Stress related transactions between person and environment. In: Dervin, L.A., Lewis, M. (eds.) *Perspectives in Interpersonal Psychology*. New York, NY: Plenum.

Lewin, K. (1951) *Field Theory in Social Science*. New York, NY: Harper and Row.

Marsh, G., Davis, M., Igoe, J. (in press) Family Community Health

McGee, G.K. (1993) Making performance appraisals a positive experience. *Nursing Management*; 23, 36–37.

News (1998) DoH figures confirm recruitment problems. *Nursing Standard*; 12; 30, 6.

Nolan, M., Brown, J., Naughton, M. et al (1998) Evidence-based care: can we overcome the barriers? *British Journal of Nursing*; 7: 17, 1044–1048.

Peters, T. (1988) *Thriving on Chaos: Handbook for Management Revolution*. New York, NY: Macmillan.

Pryjmachuk, S. (1996) Pragmatism and change: some implications for nurses, nurse managers and nursing. *Journal of Nursing Management*; 4, 201–205.

Salvage, J. (1984) *The Politics of Nursing*. London: Heinemann Nursing.

Sullivan, E.J., Decker, P.J. (1997) *Effective Leadership and Management in Nursing.* (4th edition) Harlow, England: Addison-Wesley.

Timpson, J. (1996) Towards an understanding of the human resource in the context of change in the NHS: economic sense versus cultural sensibilities. *Journal of Nursing Management*; 4, 315–324.

Toffler, A. (1973) *Future Shock.* London: Pan Books.

United Kingdom Central Council for Nursing, Midwifery and Health Visiting (1996) *Initial Position Statement on Clinical Supervision in Nursing and Health Visiting.* London: UKCC.

Walsh, M. (1997) Perceptions of barriers to implementing research. *Nursing Standard*; 11: 19, 34–37.

Walsh, M., Ford, P. (1989) *Nursing Rituals.* London: Butterworth Heinemann.

Watson, S. (1998) Trusts reject applicants despite staffing crisis. *Nursing Standard*; 12: 50, 8.

Williams, S., Michie, S., Pattani, S. (1998) *Improving the Health of the Workforce: Report of the Partnership on the Health of the NHS Workforce.* Nuffield Trust Report. London: Nuffield Trust.

Wright, S., Elliot, M., Schofield, H. (1997) A network approach to clinical supervision. *Nursing Standard*; 11: 18, 39–41.

Wright, S. (1998) *Changing Nursing Practice.* London: Edward Arnold.

6 Researching clinical supervision

Robert McSherry

In this chapter I will consider the need for clinical supervision in light of rising public expectation and patient dependency and the growing need to support healthcare professions within the healthcare environment during this demanding and stressful period. Advice will be offered on how research and the research process may be used to assist with the implementation and evaluation of clinical supervision within the clinical area. Within this section some of the key issues surrounding the use of research to underpin the development and evaluation of clinical supervision will be explored. Finally, the problems of attribution will be discussed. To help clarify the key issues within this chapter, reflective activities, case studies and examples of good practice from my experience will be used.

WHY THE NEED FOR CLINICAL SUPERVISION: RISING EXPECTATIONS, INCREASING PATIENT DEPENDENCY AND THE ABILITY TO SUPPORT STAFF

As already explained in Chapter 1, clinical supervision is about establishing a process whereby practitioners and skilled supervisors meet to reflect on both positive and negative practices (clinical, educational or managerial) in the pursuit of improving practice and increasing professional understanding (Kohner, 1994; Faugier and Butterworth, 1994; UKCC, 1996).

Activity 1: Contributing factors that indicate the need for implementing and evaluating clinical supervision within your clinical setting

As a ward manager, senior or junior qualified nurse, pause and reflect for a moment on the current healthcare environment and note down all the contributing factors that indicate the need for implementing and evaluating clinical supervision within your clinical setting.

One only has to read the many nursing journals and turn to the jobs pages to see that currently nursing (including midwifery and health visiting) is experiencing great pressures in recruitment and selection, and in the retention of staff. These pressures seem to have developed over the past 10 years following the introduction of several significant government reforms. These Department of Health publications include the white paper, *Working for Patients* (1989), *The Patients Charter: Raising the Standard* (1992), *The Code on Openness in the NHS* (1997) and, latterly, *The New NHS: Modern, Dependable* (1998).

These reforms have been directed towards increasing efficiency and effectiveness along with the standards and quality of healthcare provision, while increasing the public's awareness of access to healthcare. The struggle for improved standards and quality of care within an efficient and effective NHS has witnessed the introduction of advanced supporting technology and surgical interventions, for example, pressure-relieving equipment and minimal invasive surgery. This means that an individual patient's average length of stay in hospital for some major operations and medical treatment has been markedly reduced, while requests for information have increased, placing immense pressure on staff to meet these demands.

The reduction in patients' stays is exacerbated by the fact that patient dependency is rising due to demographic changes within society. According to the Department of Health *Health of the Nation* document, between '1981 and 1989 the number of people aged 75–84 has risen by 16%, and those 85 and over by 39%' (Department of Health, 1993); a phenomenon predicted to continue well into the 21st century.

Increased life expectancy means that patients who are admitted onto acute medical, surgical, orthopaedic and elderly care wards and into the community have far more multiple pathologies, resulting in complex social circumstances and requiring greater support in a shorter period of time from the health professionals around them. If this is true, it becomes even more imperative for nurses (indeed, all health professionals) to work in an environment that offers support and advice to reduce the stresses experienced by staff. Clinical supervision offers the opportunity to assist with this challenge (see Chapter 2).

While clinical supervision is 'claimed to be professionally beneficial. It must also protect the patient or client as it assists the development of better skills and attitudes' (Darley, 1996). If this is correct, clinical supervision could be seen to be an essential tool in aiding the reduction of clinical risks and promoting clinical effectiveness.

The whole process of clinical supervision fits nicely into the current system of 'clinical governance', which 'can best be summarised as a protective mechanism (umbrella) for both the public and healthcare professionals, ensuring that their local hospitals and community trusts are actively developing structures to improve the quality of care in the hope of preventing any recurrence of the Bristol Case, 1998' (McSherry and Haddock, 1999).

Clinical supervision is a key component of clinical governance in that it allows staff 'protected time out' to reflect on the care offered or professional issues pertinent to the individual under the guidance of a supervisor. This in turn promotes better standards and quality of care, as will be highlighted when looking at attribution.

Activity I feedback

Summary of contributing factors that indicate the need for implementing and evaluating clinical supervision within your clinical setting:

▶ Difficulties with recruitment, selection and retention of registered nurses.

▶ Government reforms directed towards improving the quality and standards of care along with the efficiency and effectiveness of the NHS.

▶ Rising patient and carer expectations.

▶ Advances in information technology.

▶ Demographic changes:

Increased life expectancy

Increasing numbers of older people.

Greater patient dependencies.

In order to meet the above changes in healthcare and to support the healthcare staff in doing so, the establishment of a system of clinical supervision that is appropriate and relevant to each hospital or community trust, ward, department or individual is essential.

USING RESEARCH AND THE RESEARCH PROCESS TO DEVELOP AND EVALUATE CLINICAL SUPERVISION

Before discussing how research and the research process may help you to develop and evaluate a strategy or system of clinical supervision within your clinical or work area, it is important that you understand what research and the research process are and why we need research.

Case study 1: The importance of research and the research process in supporting the development of patient care

Clare is a senior staff nurse working on a busy acute medical ward for the older person. While undertaking the role of supervisor during an allocated clinical supervision session for a junior colleague, the junior member of staff (who has had no research experience) asks Clare why one of her patients has been asked to participate in some research on the ward that the consultant is coordinating.

Let us consider how Clare may answer the question so that the junior member of staff may understand what research and the research process are and their importance in promoting quality standards of care.

In order to answer the above question Clare may draw Fig 6.1, summarising the key points supporting the need for research within the clinical area.

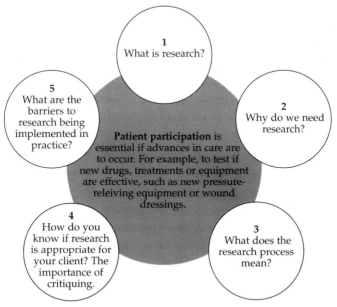

Fig 6.1 Patient participation and the need for research awareness

Clare may start answering the question by explaining to her junior colleague that the participation of patients, carers and healthcare professionals in research is essential if advances in care are to occur. Examples would be testing if new drugs, treatments or equipment are effective, such as the introduction of new pressure-relieving equipment or wound dressings. Clare may briefly point out to her supervisee the importance of the following in order for the supervisee to use research to support practice:

▶ What is meant by the term 'research'?

▶ Why do we need it?

▶ How is research conducted? (The importance of critical appraisal skills.)

▶ What prevents it from being implemented?

The following explanations may be offered along with references for further reading. An important point of supervision is that the supervisee learns from their experience and they may have to do some extra practice or professional development in order to address any issues raised.

What is research?

Clare may reinforce to her supervisee that research is 'an attempt to increase the sum of what is known, usually referred to as a body of knowledge, by the discovery of new facts or relationships, through the process of systematic scientific enquiry' (Macleod-Clarke and Hockey, 1989). Research is about developing new practices and testing out old ones, such as why we continue to starve patients from midnight, when sufficient research is available to suggest otherwise. Clare may summarise what research is by stressing its importance in improving the standard and quality of nursing care, hence why her patient may have been asked to participate in some research in the clinical area.

Why do we need research?

Clare may inform her supervisee that following the publication of the 'Briggs Report' (1972), which stated that 'nursing should become a research-based profession', it would appear that Britain's nurses have been overcome by a surge in the desire to increase their understanding and utilisation of research. As a result, large amounts of 'textual' and 'article' materials are available on the topics of 'Nursing Research' and 'The Research Process', which can be categorised into the following:

▶ 'Defining Research' – Chandler (1988); Nolan and Behi (1995).

▶ 'Nursing Research and Practice' – Linderman (1988).

▶ 'Advantages and Disadvantages of Qualitative and Quantitative Research' – Thurston and Burt (1990); Clarke (1994).

▶ 'Ethical and Moral Dilemmas in Research' – Clarke (1994).

The availability of articles and material seems to be endless, demonstrating a proliferation of activity to justify the need for a 'research-based approach to practice' and the instigation of 'evidence-based care'.

According to Hunt (1987), nursing research has only developed in Britain over the past 15 years. Therefore 'it is still in an infantile state in research terms'. In spite of this, considerable claims have been made that nursing research is largely incomprehensible, unread and unused by practising nurses. Perhaps this is a reason why few nurses have started to use research in practice. This is a problem that continues to exist today, ensuring that nursing becomes research-focused, and differentiating between those activities that are scientific-based and those from previous experiences or common sense (McSherry, 1997).

Research is about generating new knowledge and testing existing knowledge, and is essential for improving the standards and quality of patient care. Research carried out by scientists generates knowledge more systematically and rigorously than non-scientists who are simply going about the business of everyday life. The pressure facing many nurses is to develop skills, knowledge and competencies to be able to practise nursing as a 'scientific-based' profession.

Keteflan (1975), Buckenham and McGrath (1983) and Chandler (1988) support the notion that nursing research is the pathway through which professionalism can be pursued. Professionalism and professional effectiveness may be achieved when 'individuals have learned to maximise their knowledge and skills and are in a 'learning and practice' environment that also maximises the use of their ability' (Deane and Campbell, 1985). Deane and Campbell's work surrounding nursing research and the achievement of professionalism seems to be positive and supports the need for research.

The UKCC Code of Professional Conduct (1992) states that 'each trained member is meant to assume responsibility for his/her own continual education and development of practice'. Clark and Hockey's (1979) evidence seems to support the UKCC statement by suggesting that nurses can use relevant research findings, if such findings are available; and the impression obtained from current research literature, such as LoBiondo-Wood and Harber (1990), is that such findings are available and provide indicators for practice. Clare may reinforce to her junior colleague that it is all very well knowing about what research is and why we need research to support the development of practice, but it is also important to understand how research is performed.

What is the research process?

The research process is defined as 'a framework made up of a sequence of logical steps within which research is carried out. It provides a chronological list of the tasks to be done in order to complete successfully a research project. The list can be used as headings in writing up your research report' (Parahoo and Reid, 1988). The research process (framework) as offered by Hawthorne (1983), Cormack (1996) and Crombie (1997) provides a foundation on which to build critical appraisal skills essential for developing or examining any research paper or project.

How do you know if research is appropriate for your client? The importance of critiquing

The importance of critical appraisal and its application to healthcare practice is well documented in the literature (Crombie, 1997; Parahoo and Reid, 1988; McSherry, 1997) in achieving good standards and quality care when basing practice around sound research evidence. However, a fundamental issue facing many nurses, midwives and health visitors is not having the knowledge, skills or experience to critique effectively. The literature offered by Crombie (1996), Sackett et al (1997) and Swage (1998) seems to suggest that critical appraisal is about considering the relevance of a research question, evaluating the evidence collected to answer the question, and assessing the effectiveness of the conclusion and recommendation of the evidence.

Put simply, it is about systematically reviewing and questioning the stages of the research process, that is title and abstract, introduction/literature review, methods, results, discussions and recommendations and asking the following:

▶ Is the research of interest?

▶ Why was it done?

▶ How was it performed?

▶ What did it show?

▶ What is the possible implication for your practice?

▶ What next? Information only, uninteresting or support practice.

Adapted from Crombie (1997).

Barriers to research utilisation

Hunt's (1987) study on 'Indicators for nursing practice: the use of research findings' demonstrated five reasons to account for the slow uptake of nurses using research, as follows:

▶ Nurses do not know about research findings.

▶ Nurses do not understand the research process and findings.

▶ Nurses do not believe research findings.

▶ Nurses do not know how to apply the research findings.

▶ Nurses are not allowed to use the research findings.

Greenwood (1984) supports Hunt's findings by stating that nurses are slow off the mark in using research to enhance patient care. In the 'Position Paper on Nursing Research', Greenwood purports another two factors why research is not being used; factors that are easy to see but are always being overlooked. 'Clinically nurses do not perceive research findings as relevant to their practice; they do not perceive them as relevant to their practice because frequently they are not relevant' (1984). Greenwood's paper may be accurate in stating that nurses' perceptions of research, and the relevance of the research, may influence the individual nurse's ability to 'understand' and 'utilise' research findings in practice. Another fundamental phenomenon seems to emerge, missed from Hunt's (1987), Greenwood's (1984) and much other recent literature, and that is 'pressure'. McSherry (1997) and Cohen and Manion (1985) suggest that while most nurses do apply a problem-solving approach to their practice, the knowledge they use is often a combination of rituals and tradition. This in turn creates a problem when considering that the majority of nurses have had little, if any, training on the research process and how to introduce it (McSherry, 1997).

Case study 1 feedback

Clare may summarise to her supervisee that in order for her to understand why one of her patients has been asked to participate in some research on the ward, the following aspects associated with research need to be addressed:

▶ What is research?

▶ Why do we need research?

▶ What is the research process?

▶ How do you know if research is appropriate for your client? (The importance of critiquing.)

▶ Barriers to research utilisation.

Suggested further reading

Crombie, I. (1997) *The Pocket Guide to Critical Appraisal*. London: British Medical Journal Publishing Group.

Linderman, C.B. (1988) Research in practice: the role of the staff nurse. *Applied Nursing Research*; 1: 1, 5–7.

LoBiondo-Wood, G., Harber, J. (1990) *Nursing Research: Methods, Critical Appraisal and Utilisation*. Toronto: The CV Mosby Company.

McSherry, R., Haddock, J. (1999) Evidence-based healthcare: its place within clinical governance. *British Journal of Nursing*; 8: 2, 113–117.

Nolan, M., Behi, R. (1995) What is research? Some definitions and dilemmas. *British Journal of Nursing*; 4: 2, 111–115

RESEARCH SUPPORTING THE DEVELOPMENT OF CLINICAL SUPERVISION

As identified, research is essential in developing and testing new and existing skills and knowledge in a systematic and scientific way. This is usually referred to as the 'research process', offering a sequential or chronological set of stages fundamental to either an individual or organisation in establishing or evaluating a research project. In addition, the research framework is an allele to developing critical thinking and appraisal skills – essential attributes for all healthcare professionals in the pursuit of evidence-based care and standards of clinical excellence. Research plays an important part in promoting individual and professional development along with improving the standards and quality of patient care by the generation and testing of new and existing rituals, traditions and practices.

Case study 2: How research may support the introduction of clinical supervision within your ward/clinical area

As a senior sister/charge nurse you have been informed that your hospital/nursing home or community trust supports the concept of clinical supervision and wants to see a strategy for achieving this for all grades of staff under your management.

Think about how research and the research process may aid you in carrying out the above request.

The starting point is to use research and the research process to help you and your colleagues develop a realistic and simple strategy that supports the clinical area and staff needs. This will only be achieved by involving staff and informing them about the rationale and benefits for clinical supervision. Remember that in order to achieve new initiatives successfully, realistic and flexible time and personnel management are essential. Staff ownership, participation and encouragement all need to be accounted for in a simple but reliable action plan that is shared, owned and, most importantly, agreed by all (where possible). Fig 6.2 offers a simple 10-step guide to supporting the implementation and evaluation of clinical supervision. This will be discussed later in more detail. The shaded areas 1–6 support the implementation processes of clinical supervision and the white areas 7–10 support the evaluation process.

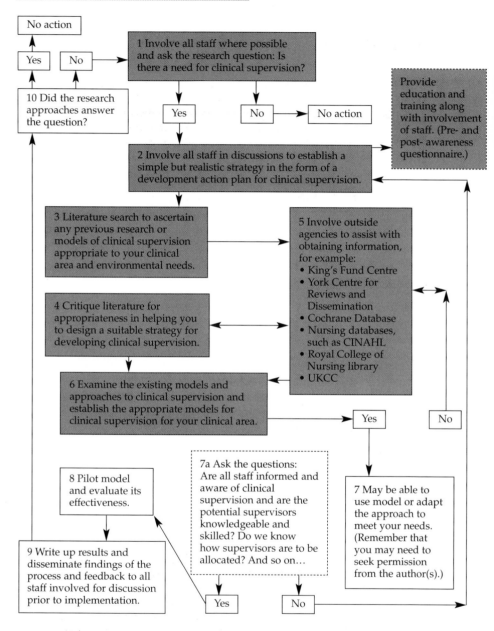

Fig 6.2 Using the research process to aid the implementation of clinical supervision

A guide to implementation of clinical supervision

The starting point for successful implementation of any new initiative or innovation within the clinical area is communicating and sharing your idea with colleagues. The question that needs addressing is whether you have the backing and support of your colleagues for introducing clinical supervision. If staff are in favour, introduce shared ownership of the project. In this way, the allocation of key roles and responsibilities, such as those described below, can be instigated.

Literature searching (Step 4)

There are many places that may be willing to offer support to aid you with the introduction of clinical supervision. However, it is important to explore all possible avenues in order to enhance the quality of your work.

Sources of help

- ▶ King's Fund Centre;
- ▶ local hospital library (books/journals);
- ▶ data search CINAHL;
- ▶ the internet;
- ▶ United Kingdom Central Council;
- ▶ other trust wards using clinical supervision;
- ▶ practice development centres;
- ▶ clinical audit departments;
- ▶ research departments;
- ▶ local universities.

Critiquing the literature (Step 5)

It is essential that the information obtained be critiqued for its usefulness and effectiveness in meeting your unique set of clinical needs. An examination of the existing models and literature (Step 6) is essential in establishing a model or system of clinical supervision that best fits your needs. A reflection on how other professional groups or organisations have orchestrated a system of clinical supervision is fundamental in helping you promote best practices and prevent mistakes. Some practical considerations to draw from the examination of the information associated with implementing clinical supervision are described below.

Selection of supervisors and education of staff (Step 7a)

The selection and preparation of supervisors is a highly important issue when looking at successfully implementing clinical supervision. The following issues should be taken into account:

▶ The number of supervisees to supervisors.

▶ Do you have a register of supervisors?

▶ How are supervisors linked to supervisees?

▶ How are the supervisors to be prepared for the role?

These are all areas that may be addressed when exploring the literature.

Many hospitals and community trusts are establishing their own in-house training or collaborating with local universities to establish educational programmes relating to informing staff about clinical supervision or for the training of supervisors. Many different approaches may be adopted, ranging from formal modular-based programmes to individual study days. What is most important when choosing a training programme is to establish what best meets your requirements.

Resources and environmental issues

The most fundamental question that needs asking is whether the implementation of clinical supervision can be accommodated given the existing workload and skill mix. If the answer is no, then the question of resources may need to be taken to managers for guidance and support. Practical issues that need to be addressed include the nature of supervision (one-to-one or group), the frequency of the sessions (monthly, twice-yearly or on request), where the sessions will take place and who is responsible for booking and informing staff members about cancellation.

The processes of clinical supervision

Key points to consider include:

▶ The boundaries to confidentiality – if either party feels an issue cannot be kept within the confinement of a session, for example in breach of the code of professional conduct, breaking the law and so on.

▶ What will happen if either party fails to keep an appointment, feels unhappy with the quality of the clinical supervision or feels the need for outside support to resolve an issue.

These limits or boundaries need to be highlighted and ground rules agreed.

Documentation

With the rising numbers of litigation cases within healthcare, it is imperative that appropriate structures for monitoring and evaluating clinical supervision are created. These will assist in demonstrating the possible benefits of clinical supervision for an individual, profession or healthcare organisation. (See section on attribution.)

The documentation may be varied to capture key aspects associated with the delivery and evaluation of clinical supervision, and could include the following:

▶ Register of supervisors.

▶ Form to record evidence of training and education.

▶ Contract/ground rules form to be completed on first session and evaluated periodically.

▶ Supervisors' and supervisees' individual records.

▶ Auditing forms showing occurrence of sessions.

The issue of who keeps the records and receives auditing documentation will need to be agreed.

As identified, all practical issues need to be addressed in order to ensure that staff are aware of what it is you are aiming to achieve when introducing clinical supervision. Other similar wards or units may have already overcome many of the practical issues, hence the importance of researching the topic efficiently and effectively.

Additional practical considerations

The two boxes with dotted outlines in Fig 6.2 contain practical questions that may need answering in order to ensure that the project is developed successfully. For example, it may be worth establishing a baseline assessment of staff awareness of clinical supervision early on in the process, in order to evaluate the effectiveness of education and training or to promote awareness, before leaping into developing a model/system of clinical supervision.

What might a baseline questionnaire look like?

As previously indicated, it is fundamentally important to stress the need to assess, plan, implement and evaluate an appropriate model of clinical supervision that best meets with your underlying philosophy, staff attitude and culture on the ward or within the organisation. The design and content of your initial research will be interdependent on many factors, such as time, finance, resources, staff interest and so on. The following simple questionnaire may serve as a baseline.

CLINICAL SUPERVISION AWARENESS QUESTIONAIRE

Please tick the appropriate boxes and feel free to add comments.

Office use

Q1: Do you know what clinical supervision is?

          Yes ☐   No ☐   1   2

If yes, please state here:

Q2: Have you any previous training in relation to clinical supervision?

          Yes ☐   No ☐   1   2

If yes, please state here:

Q3: Do you feel you need more information about clinical supervision?

          Yes ☐   No ☐   1   2

If yes, please state here:

Q4: If clinical supervision was introduced tomorrow would you feel confident in carrying it out?

          Yes ☐   No ☐   1   2

Q5: Length qualified   0–1 year ☐   1

                    2–3 years ☐   2

                    4–5 years ☐   3

                    6 years or more ☐   4

Q6: Are you a qualified or unqualified member of staff?

Qualified ☐   Unqualified ☐   1   2

Thank you for your help.

Fig 6.3 Clinical supervision awareness questionnaire

Presenting feedback of results

The example below is taken from the author's experiences of helping staff to introduce clinical supervision within a large medical directorate while working as Practice Development Advisor (PDA). The results demonstrated for this acute medical ward that the staff required education and training in order to promote awareness before devising a strategy for implementation of clinical supervision.

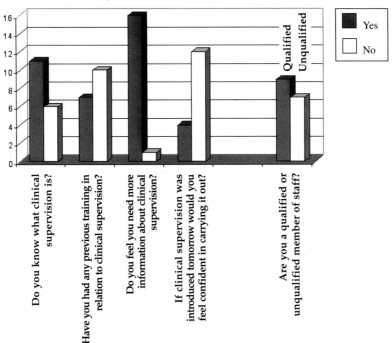

Clinical supervision awareness questionnaire

Fig 6.4 Clinical supervision awareness questionnaire responses

The numerical data is complemented by the comments requested under each of the questions. Examples of comments include:

Q2: Have you had any previous training in relation to clinical supervision?

'A long time ago. Two years left me with more questions than answers.'

'Very brief introduction and description during training.'

Q3: Do you feel you need more information about clinical supervision?

'How to instigate it.'

'The role of the supervisor, i.e. is it a listening role or an advisory role?'

What might a development plan look like?

Step 2 (Fig 6.2) suggests that a simple and easy-to-use framework be written to form the basis of a developmental plan for implementing and evaluating clinical supervision within the clinical area. An example of how this might look and how it could be linked to the step-by-step guide is shown below.

TABLE 6.1 EXAMPLE OF A DEVELOPMENT PLAN

Start date	Topic for investigation	Action required	By who?	When?
	(Step 1) Establish research question/ reasons for and against clinical supervision within your area or organisation.	Consult staff and establish level of support **(Step 2)**. Establish current staff awareness of clinical supervision.		
	(Step 3) Literature search.	Consult external agencies for information. Search data-bases, e.g. CINAHL **(Step 2)**.		
	(Step 4) Critique the literature.	Review the literature/ information by examining existing models for their appropriateness in helping to meet your needs **(Step 6)**. Consider practical issues, such as education and training, selection of supervisors and so on.		

Start date	Topic for investigation	Action required	By who?	When?
	(Step 7) Devise model of clinical supervision for your area.	Involve all staff. Ensure all supervisors and staff are adequately trained. Set start date (may choose to pilot first). Pay attention to clinical issues, such as: • time out • rostering • privacy • supervision structure		

Case study 2 feedback

Although it appears simple, the above development plan has actually consolidated the implementation phase of Fig 6.2 and offers a step-by-step guide to using research to support the introduction of clinical supervision into your clinical area.

Key words to remember are:

▶ consultation

▶ communication

▶ commitment

▶ simplicity

▶ staff involvement

▶ shared ownership

▶ flexibility

▶ allow time

In summary, case study 2 illustrates how the research process offers a flexible and systematic framework to implementing clinical supervision by facilitating a phased approach. This becomes evident by using the key headings associated with any research project. For example:

▶ Identify problem or ask question.

▶ Do literature search.

▶ Critique the literature.

▶ Devise method of implementation.

It would be unwise and more time consuming to do a literature search without first establishing the motivation and commitment of staff behind the concept. By posing a research question or rationale for the implementation of clinical supervision within your clinical area, the whole process of literature searching becomes easier and less time consuming because you may already have an idea of the style of supervision for your setting. Examples include group supervision for an outpatient department, individual supervision for clinical nurse specialists and so on. The remainder of this chapter concentrates on evaluation of clinical supervision and the issues associated with attribution.

EVALUATING CLINICAL SUPERVISION

Steps 8–10 of Fig 6.2 may be concerned with the introduction of clinical supervision after piloting a model/system or after a formal period of introduction. In order to achieve the evaluation successfully it is imperative to describe how the various approaches to research (qualitative or quantitative) may be allied to this process.

The various approaches to research

Clinical supervision, although a relatively new concept to nursing (but not midwifery), has seen a proliferation in research aimed at defining and establishing the benefits of the concept at national and local levels (Faugier and Butterworth, 1994; Webb, 1997; Yegdich, 1998; Lewis, 1998; Bishop, 1998). The difficulty that many clinical staff, educationalists and academics seem to have is in rationalising how such a diverse and complex concept, involving feelings, attitudes, reflexivity and critical analysis of an individual's clinical, professional and personal practices, can be measured, let alone evaluated, by using research.

The starting point in overcoming this issue is to define the various approaches to research, preceded by an example of how they unite in aiding the evaluation of Proctor's model of clinical supervision (1992). According to the literature offered by Seers (1994), Gilbert (1994) and Cormack (1996) there are two common ways by which research can be approached – 'quantitative' or 'qualitative'. Quantitative research is a more systematic, formal or objective approach associated with using numerical and statistical data in the pursuit of answering questions about the world. The research usually attempts to answer questions associated with frequency or occurrences in order to make reliable and valid measures of a concept, and thus produces results that can be generalised. This is typically why quantitative research is seen to test theories (a deductive approach), and uses theories as its starting point. The types of research designs covered are often experimental, attitudinal or survey designs.

Question: Is there any evidence of this approach being used to support the implementation or evaluation of clinical supervision?

Answer: Yes.

Bishop (1998) presented a paper outlining the results of a large survey of trust nurse executive's feedback on how clinical supervision was or was not progressing in their organisation. Of the 410 questionnaires distributed, 273 were returned (67% return rate).

For more information read: Bishop, V. (1998) Clinical supervision: what's going on? Results of a questionnaire. *Nursing Times*; 94: 18, 50–53.

Qualitative research, on the other hand, is a more subjective approach using life experiences, personal accounts, diaries or observational practices of a given phenomenon or event in order to understand the meaning behind the occurrence. Unlike quantitative research, qualitative research encourages the development of theories (inductive approach) from the observations of individual or group practices.

The types of research designs covered are often focus groups, semi-structured interviews or observational practices.

Question: Is there any evidence of this approach being used to support the implementation or evaluation of clinical supervision?

Answer: Yes.

Sloan's (1998) paper demonstrates the use of focus groups as a data collection method, detailing how the group discussion was analysed, resulting with the relevant 'good characteristics' of a clinical supervisor from the supervisee's perspective.

For more information read:

Sloan, G. (1998) Focus group interview: defining clinical supervision. *Nursing Standard*; 12: 42, 40–43.

The articles offered by Bishop and Sloan successfully demonstrate how the various approaches to research can aid the evaluation of key aspects associated with clinical supervision within the healthcare setting. Is it possible to use research to assist with the evaluation of a model of clinical supervision?

Let us explore this concept in a little more depth with reference to Proctor's model of clinical supervision (1992) (Fig 6.5). According to Proctor's model, clinical supervision has three interwoven parts that promote fundamental benefits to the individual, organisation and profession.

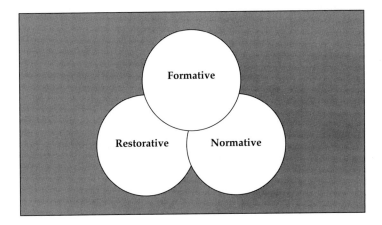

Fig 6.5 Proctor's model of clinical supervision

Key elements associated with Proctor's model

▶ *Formative* or 'educational' role, associated with the education and training of the supervisee, perhaps linked to skills and understanding of clinical practices. The uses of reflective practice on both positive and negative provisions of care are nurtured.

▶ *Restorative*, the 'supportive' role, 'relating to the way in which practitioners are able to put into perspective the stresses and strains of working in an area where intimate interactions with clients form the basis of work' (Darley, 1996).

▶ *Normative*, or 'quality standards', 'overseeing the quality of professional practice' (Lewis, 1998).

On initial inspection of Procter's model it would seem extremely difficult to associate either a qualitative or quantitative approach to evaluating a strategy of clinical supervision. This is especially evident when dealing with such diverse and complex issues as staff attitudes, reflective practice, standards, quality outcomes and professional support. How can you measure the learning or changes in professional and clinical practices of such a confidential and private relationship between either two individuals or a group of individuals?

The answer to the above dilemma seems to be by combining qualitative and quantitative research methods, known as 'triangulation'. 'Knowing a single landmark only locates one somewhere along a line in a direction from the landmark, whereas with two landmarks one can take bearings on both and locate oneself at their intersection' (Fielding and Fielding, 1986).

It may be argued that 'in research, if diverse kinds of data support the same conclusions, confidence in it is increased' (Fielding and Fielding, 1986). This can be essential if you are to provide managers with concrete evidence on how effective or ineffective clinical supervision may be for your ward, outpatient department or healthcare organisation.

By taking the following approach, and using perhaps small focus groups of staff to establish their current level of knowledge and awareness of clinical supervision, the responses could be seen to be reflective of the organisational culture and representative of staff attitudes. A quantitative questionnaire may be designed using the key themes and distributed to an entire ward or organisation in the hope of establishing a baseline of overall staff awareness and knowledge, and the benefits of clinical supervision.

Case study 3: Using a combination of research methods to evaluate Proctor's model

As a senior sister/charge nurse of an acute medical ward you would like to evaluate your current system of clinical supervision (based on Proctor's model). Determine what information you will need to obtain and how best to present the results to managers.

What information do I need to obtain?

The following are indicators of the sort of information that you might collect in order to demonstrate the effectiveness of clinical supervision:

- Number of staff who have had training and nature of training.
- Number of trained supervisors.
- Who are the supervisors?
- What is staff awareness of clinical supervision?
- Issues associated with venues, frequency of supervision sessions, cancellation of sessions.
- How do staff feel about receiving clinical supervision?
- Has the level of staff sickness increased or decreased?
- What are staff attitudes on the ward?
- Do staff feel supported?
- Has the level of incident reporting or patient complaints or patient satisfaction improved?

Using small focus groups, semi-structured or structured interviews may capture information associated with staff attitudes, frequency of clinical supervision sessions and any other issues that staff may have about venues, support, improved morale or the perceived benefits of clinical supervision.

Alternatively, a questionnaire may be designed that would be completed after the focus groups have met or distributed at the same time as running the groups in order to reinforce the findings.

A simple questionnaire may look something like the following:

CLINICAL SUPERVISION QUESTIONNAIRE

Please tick the appropriate box.

All information will be treated in strictest confidence and anonymity will be maintained

Q1: Do you currently receive clinical supervision?   Yes ☐   No ☐

Comments:

Q2: Do you have an identified supervisor?   Yes ☐   No ☐

Comments:

Q3: What form does your supervision take?
(You may tick more than one box)

Planned ☐

Informal chats ☐

One-to-one ☐

Peer ☐

Group ☐

Other. Please state...

Q4: How many clinical supervision sessions have you had to date?
Total ....

Q5: Have you benefited from receiving clinical supervision?

Comments:

Q6: Have you any negative experiences of clinical supervision?

Comments:

Q7: What did you find useful to discuss in the clinical supervision session?

Comments:

Q8: Have you had any sessions cancelled?

Comments:

Q9: Are you currently supervising a colleague?   Yes ☐   No ☐

Q10: Do you have any concerns or anxieties about being a supervisor?

Comments:

Q11: Do you have any concerns or anxieties about being supervised?

Comments:

Q12: Do you feel that you have sufficient knowledge and skills to supervise another colleague?

Comments:

Are you

Qualified? ☐

Unqualified? ☐

If qualified, please answer the following:

Please state your grade . . . .

Length qualified . . . .

Numbers of supervisees . . . .

Ward . . . .   Directorate . . . .

Thank you for your help. Please return to . . . .

Fig 6.6 Example of a simple questionnaire

Please note that this questionnaire is only shown as a guide. For a more rigorous and detailed questionnaire it would be advisable to enlist the help of experts, especially in the design and ordering of questions.

Data analysis

This is a highly important aspect in preparing feedback for staff or management. You will need to ensure that you are adequately prepared to interpret and present the results in a format that best suits your ward and organisational needs. The results of the above questionnaire could be presented in the form of graphs or pie charts, supported with factual qualitative data taken from the subjects' comments.

A final point to remember is that using the appropriate research approach(es) with the relevant methods (individual or combined) will assist in providing you with a more valid and reliable set of results related to the model of clinical supervision of your choice. Always seek professional advice if you are unsure. Failing to take advice at this important stage may invalidate your results and any future evaluations.

Case study 3 feedback

From this case study it becomes clear that either a single qualitative or quantitative approach, using one or more methods, or a combined approach (triangulation, using several methods) may be used to examine the whole concept of clinical supervision.

Although not explicit in the case example, it could be fair to suggest that by concentrating on staff educational needs and awareness, we are examining the formative aspect of Proctor's model. Likewise, looking at staff attitudes towards giving and receiving clinical supervision relates to the restorative function of the model. Finally, any evidence of a reduction in incident reporting, staff sickness or patient complaints or an increase in levels of satisfaction may be an indicator of the quality effect it is having on the ward and organisation.

In essence, according to White et al (1998), an evaluation of the effectiveness of clinical supervision should be central to three areas: structure, process and outcomes. The structure perhaps refers to the frequency, environment and location of a clinical supervision session. The process associated with the model and the way you deliver clinical supervision are contracts established, ground rules set and documentation written. Outcomes related to the potential benefits of supervision at an individual, personal and professional level are essential as this last section on attribution demonstrates.

There are many important things to remember when doing research, which can help to elicit a successful outcome.

▶ Always seek management approval and communicate your interests.

▶ Seek approval from your peers and ward staff. (Involve them in the process.)

▶ Ensure staff confidentiality and anonymity are maintained.

▶ Send the questionnaire with a stamped addressed envelope and letter of explanation.

▶ Allow sufficient time for the questionnaire to be returned.

▶ Be specific with wording on the questionnaire.

THE PROBLEMS OF ATTRIBUTION

According to Collins English Dictionary, attribution is 'a characteristic or quality of a person or thing' (Collins, 1987). The dilemma facing many hospital and community trust or healthcare organisations is in establishing an efficient and effective system or framework to evaluate the effectiveness and outcomes associated with such a complex concept as clinical supervision.

On initial inspection of the current literature surrounding clinical supervision, it would be easy to suggest that attribution is interdependent on the model in use. For example, Proctor's model should concentrate on the formative, restorative and normative elements attributed to clinical supervision. The evaluation would focus on issues such as:

▶ Formative – education, training, understanding.

▶ Restorative – supporting structures, alleviating staff stresses.

▶ Normative – patient and staff satisfaction and standards/quality and clinical risk issues.

The reality of achieving a robust evaluation of such a diverse and complex concept as clinical supervision is and will remain very difficult. This is because the concept deals with staff attitudes and feelings that are entwined into so many compounding organisational and environmental variables: skill mix, patient dependency, case loads, length of stay, bed numbers and so on, making it hard to formulate and refine research to one specific target area.

Question: Has any research or literature been written highlighting the potential benefits of using clinical supervision?

Answer: Yes.

According to recent research studies and literature (Kohner, 1994; Fowler, 1995; Darley, 1996; Sloan, 1998; White et al, 1998), the benefits of clinical supervision seem to be categorised into three prominent areas, as follows:

▶ individual

▶ organisational

▶ professional

Individual

According to Darley (1996), by encouraging nurses to reflect on their own clinical practices – the key mechanism of clinical supervision – this may foster a better understanding of individual, professional and employment accountability. This may therefore 'make a serious contribution to risk management strategies' (Darley, 1996) and the introduction of evidence-based care and the principles of clinical governance (McSherry and Haddock, 1999).

The exploratory research study offered by White et al (1998), who interviewed staff to establish the potential benefits of clinical supervision, reinforces the above by suggesting that practitioners 'welcomed the development of their confidence and self-esteem, the support they derived from peers and the sense of 'actually taking responsibility' for their own practice' (White et al, 1998).

Organisational

The literature offered by White et al (1998) suggests that the introduction of clinical supervision may enhance staff morale and be an incentive to recruiting staff because staff are able to feel supported and listened to. Darley (1996) feels that an effective evaluation of clinical supervision should demonstrate 'tangible benefits like reduced absentee levels, better take up of formal and informal education' and may even be a contributor to developing standards and quality through reflective practice on clinical incidents.

Professional

It would be fair to suggest that by having a system of clinical supervision the uniting of everyday professional and clinical practices can be developed that may, in turn, produce a more accountable, responsible and effective clinical practitioner, which must enhance the standard and quality of the profession.

Summary

While clinical supervision may offer many valuable benefits to individuals, organisations and professional bodies by reducing levels of sickness, complaints, absences and work-related injury and encouraging recruitment and retention, the realities of achieving this in today's healthcare climate, although imperative, are difficult. This is due to the recruitment and retention crisis and low staffing levels compounded by low morale and high activity.

The practical issues of staff release time, resources, facilities and cost to allow staff time out all need to be discussed and thought through in order to make clinical supervision a reality, rather than a myth.

As the UKCC suggests, and which all hospital and community healthcare trusts have a responsibility to act on, 'the UKCC endorses the establishment of clinical supervision in the interest of maintaining and improving standards of care in an often uncertain and rapidly changing health and social care environment. The UKCC commends this initiative to all practitioners, managers and those involved in negotiating contracts as an important part of strategies to promote high standards of nursing and health visiting care into the next century' (UKCC, 1996).

How can we fail to respond?

CONCLUSION

Clinical supervision is more than just a management tool to enhance standards and professional practice; it is essential in providing support to clinical staff in order to 'improve the quality of patient care' (Bishop, 1994).

Within any organisation there is a need to establish a practical understanding of supervision, to be shared by those giving and those receiving. This is about:

▶ the purpose of supervision;

▶ the process (or how supervision will be carried out);

▶ the content and focus of supervision;

▶ the relationship between supervision and management.

It is important to take into account:

▶ the needs of patients/clients;

▶ the needs of staff;

▶ the circumstances and needs of the unit;

▶ existing organisational structures;

▶ available resources;

▶ the experiences and abilities of available supervisors.

(Kohner, 1994)

In adhering to the above and using the information offered in this chapter, research may become an aid and comfort in the assessment, planning, implementation and evaluation of a strategy of clinical supervision within your clinical area.

Good luck!

REFERENCES

Abdellah, F. (1969) The nature of nursing science. *Nursing Research*; 18: 5, 390–393.

Bishop, V. (1994) Clinical supervision: what's going on? Results of a questionnaire. *Nursing Times*; 94: 18, 50–53.

Briggs, A. (1972) *Report of the Committee on Nursing*. London: HMSO.

Buckenham, E.J., McGrath, G. (1983) *The Social Reality of Nursing*. Bristol: Health Service Press.

Chandler, V.J. (1988) Science, knowledge and research: what and why for nursing. *Orthopaedic Nursing;* 7: 3, 41–44.

Clark, E., Hockey, L. (1979) Knowledge is a precious possession. *Nursing Mirror;* 152: 13, 46–49.

Clarke, J. (1994) Moral dilemmas in nursing research. *Nursing Practice;* 4: 4, 22–25.

Cohen, L., Manion, L. (1985) *Research Methods in Education.* (2nd edition) London: Routledge.

Collins, W. (1987) *Collins Universal English Dictionary.* London: William Collins Sons & Co Ltd.

Cormack, D. (1996) *The Research Process in Nursing.* London: Blackwell Science Publication.

Crombie, I. (1997) *The Pocket Guide to Critical Appraisal.* London: British Medical Journal Publishing Group.

Darley, M. (1996) Can clinical supervision improve risk management? *Health Care Risk Report;* 14: 3, 20–21.

Deane, D., Campbell, J. (1985) *Developing Professional Effectiveness in Nursing.* Virginia: Rector Publishing Company.

Department of Health (1989) *The White Paper: Working for Patients.* London: HMSO.

Department of Health (1992) *The Patients' Charter: Raising the Standard.* London: HMSO.

Department of Health (1993) *The Health of the Nation.* London: HMSO.

Department of Health (1997) *The Code of Openness in the NHS.* London: HMSO.

Department of Health (1998) *The New NHS: Modern, Dependable.* London: HMSO.

Faugier, J., Butterworth, T. (1994) *Clinical Supervision: A Position Paper.* Manchester: University of Manchester.

Fielding, G.N., Fielding, I.J. (1986) *Linking Data: Qualitative Research Methods Series.* London: Sage Publications.

Fowler, J. (1995) Nurses' perceptions of the elements of good supervision. *Nursing Times;* 91: 22, 33–37.

Gilbert, N. (1994) *Researching Social Life.* London: Sage Publications.

Greenwood, J. (1984) Nursing research: a position paper. *Journal of Advanced Nursing;* 9: 2, 77–82.

Hawthorne, P. (1983) Principles of research: a checklist. *Nursing Times;* 79: 23, 41–42.

Hunt, M. (1987) The process of translating research findings into practice. *Journal of Advanced Nursing;* 12: 5, 101–110.

Keteflan, S. (1975) Application of selected nursing research findings into practice. *Nursing Research;* 24: 2, 89–94.

Kohner, N. (1994) *Clinical Supervision: An Executive Summary.* London: King's Fund Centre.

Lewis, D. (1998) Clinical supervision for nurse lecturers. *Nursing Standard;* 12: 29, 40–42.

Linderman, C.B. (1988) Research in practice: the role of the staff nurse. *Applied Nursing Research;* 1: 1, 5–7.

LoBiondo-Wood, G., Harber, J. (1990) *Nursing Research: Methods, Critical Appraisal and Utilisation.* Toronto: The CV Mosby Company.

Macleod-Clarke, M., Hockey, J. (1989) *Further Research in Nursing.* London: Scutari Press.

McSherry, R. (1997) What do registered nurses and midwives feel and know about research? *Journal of Advanced Nursing;* 25: 6, 985–998.

McSherry, R., Haddock, J. (1999) Evidence-based health care: its place within clinical governance. *British Journal of Nursing;* 8: 2, 113–117.

Nolan, M., Behi, R. (1995) What is research? Some definitions and dilemmas. *British Journal of Nursing;* 4: 2, 111–115.

Parahoo, K., Reid, N. (1988) The research process. *Nursing Times;* 84: 40, 67–70.

Proctor, B. (1986) Supervision: a cooperative exercise in accountability. In: Marken, M., Payne, M. (eds.) *Enabling and Ensuring.* Leicester: Leicester National Youth Bureau and Council for Education and Training in Youth and Community Work.

Sackett, L.D., Rosenburg, W., Haynes, B.R. (1997) *Evidence-Based Medicine: How to Practise and Teach EBM.* London: Churchill Livingstone.

Seers, K. (1994) Qualitative and quantitative research. *Surgical Nurse*; 7: 6, 4–6.

Sloan, G. (1998) Focus group interviews: defining clinical supervision. *Nursing Standard*; 12: 42, 41–43.

Swage, T. (1998) Clinical care takes centre stage. *Nursing Times*; 94: 14, 40–41.

Thurston, N., Burt, M. (1990) Clinical nursing research and quality assurance: integration for improved patient care. *CJNA*; 6: 7, 18–23.

United Kingdom Central Council for Nursing, Midwifery and Health Visiting (1992) *Scope of Professional Practice*. London: UKCC.

United Kingdom Central Council for Nursing, Midwifery and Health Visiting (1996) *Position Statement on Clinical Supervision for Nursing and Health Visiting*. London: UKCC.

Webb, B. (1997) Auditing a clinical supervision training programme. *Nursing Standard*; 11: 11, 34–39.

White, E., Butterworth, T., Bishop, V. et al (1998) Clinical supervision: insider reports of a private world. *Journal of Advanced Nursing*; 28: 1, 185–192.

Yegdich, T. (1998) How not to do clinical supervision. *Journal of Advanced Nursing*; 28: 1, 193–202.

FURTHER READING

Clifford, C., Gough, S. (1990) *Nursing Research: A Skill-Based Introduction*. New York, NY: Prentice Hall.

Department of Health (1993) *Report of the Taskforce on the Strategy for Research in Nursing, Midwifery and Health Visiting*. London: Department of Health.

Dickoff, J., James, P., Semeradeck, J. (1975) Research part 1: a stance for nursing research – tenacity or inquiry. *Nursing Research*; 24: 2, 84–88.

Faugier, J., Butterworth, T. (1994) *Clinical Supervision: A Position Paper*. Manchester: University of Manchester.

Fawcett, J. (1980) A declaration of nursing independence: the relation of theory and research to nursing practice. *Journal of Nursing Administration;* 10: 7, 36–39.

Kohner, N. (1994) *Clinical Supervision: An Executive Summary.* London: King's Fund Centre.

Rafferty, M., Coleman, M. (1996) Educating nurses to undertake clinical supervision in practice. *Nursing Standard;* 10: 45, 38–41.

United Kingdom Central Council for Nursing, Midwifery and Health Visiting (1996) *Position Statement on Clinical Supervision for Nursing and Health Visiting.* London: UKCC.

White, E., Butterworth, T., Bishop, V. et al (1998) Clinical supervision: insider reports of a private world. *Journal of Advanced Nursing;* 28: 1, 185–192.

7 Implementing clinical supervision

Mick Ashman and Mac Macintosh

The implementation of any innovation, clinical supervision included, will be undertaken against the reality of having to continue to deliver the service. A point to keep sight of is that anything new is something extra that has to be done; the rest of the organisation's activities will not stop to allow you the time to concentrate on getting your initiative up and running. This means that the extra resources in time, money and effort will have to be found (Smith, 1995).

One of the first considerations when seeking to implement any change is to establish its magnitude from the point of view of the organisation. Dunphy and Stace (1990) describe how organisational change can be classified according to its impact on the organisation and cite four main categories:

▶ Fine tuning, which involves refining methods, policies and procedures, typically at department (or ward) level.

▶ Incremental adjustment, which involves distinct modifications to strategies, structures and management processes, but are not radical enough to be described as strategic.

▶ Modular transformation, which involves the major realignment or restructuring of departments. It may be radical but will not affect the whole of the organisation.

▶ Corporate transformation, which involves radical shifts in strategy and revolutionary changes throughout the organisation to structures, systems and procedures, to mission and core values, and to the distribution of power. An example would be the creation of a NHS trust.

In the case of the introduction of clinical supervision the change can be described in two ways. First, as an incremental adjustment, if it is being introduced either as a pilot or if departments themselves are allowed to introduce their own model. Second, the introduction of clinical supervision might be regarded as a modular transformation if a particular model is being introduced, with some urgency, throughout wards and departments. Once the scale of the change being proposed is determined consideration can be given to the change strategy.

APPROACH TO CHANGE

The value of participation in the change process was first highlighted by the work of Coch and French (1948). They were able to demonstrate that where change was imposed on employees their dissatisfaction manifested itself in such behaviours as increased absenteeism and lack of efficiency. However, if employees had a high degree of involvement in the change process, any decrease in efficiency arising out of changes in working practices was transient and there was no evidence of conflict as the change was introduced. Later commentators have highlighted the positive benefits of employee participation with respect to most aspects of management and leadership with organisations (Likert, 1961; McGregor, 1987; Pasmore and Friedlander, 1982).

Critics of the participative approach have suggested that it cannot be applied in all situations, and we can see that it would be extremely difficult to introduce modular or corporate transformation (as defined by Dunphy and Stace, 1990) with widespread employee participation. In such situations the participative approach is seen as time consuming and can result in the generation of unhelpful disagreements within the team.

Nevertheless, participation in the change process is linked to successful outcomes, and it will have the additional advantage of facilitating understanding of the change by the users. We would suggest that the principle of participation should be adopted wherever possible and only be discounted in situations where time constraints or the scale of the change would make it unfeasible.

STRATEGY

One approach to ensuring that participation occurs might be through the creation of a project team. The project team would be established to represent those affected by the innovation but at the same time would provide direction and collective leadership. While project teams cannot provide the total participation that Coch and French (1948) identified as being most effective, they can achieve a high degree of involvement through effective representation.

Clearly, the composition of this group will need some consideration but it is vital that its members are seen as representing those who will be using clinical supervision and who will be most affected by it. The group members must have three key attributes:

▶ the ability to carry through the demands of the project;

▶ the motivation and enthusiasm for the project;

▶ the confidence and support of their colleagues. This is probably the key element for an initiative such as clinical supervision, which will impact on the entire workforce.

This group may need to be supported by an external facilitator. This could be either someone who has relevant experience, having perhaps been through an implementation process in a similar organisation, or someone with a specialist interest in the field, for example someone who has been involved with clinical supervision from an educational or academic perspective.

Any decision to bring in external support would need to be taken by the group and will most likely arise in the event of the group feeling that they do not have the required skills or knowledge base to move forward.

Whether or not external support becomes part of the project group, the aims of the group, at this stage, will be to engage in the following:

▶ Establish the aims of clinical supervision for their area/directorate. Perhaps the most important first steps in the implementation of clinical supervision are to agree on what exactly it is and what you want it to do, and to establish how to communicate this in such a way that the chances of confusion and ambiguity are minimised. The potential for confusion is apparent when one looks to the literature for the answers to these questions. There are many differing views on what clinical supervision should be; sometimes these views are complementary, and sometimes they seem to be mutually exclusive. The literature makes claims about the possibilities of clinical supervision that include aspects of management, counselling, education, clinical practice and patient care, professional development, personal growth, motivation and morale (Goorapah, 1997). Clearly, it cannot be all of these. What is important to keep sight of is that any confusion over what you are trying to implement will develop into a significant barrier to success and may be the trigger that allows other problems to emerge.

▶ Based on the views of the team, the project group will be able to decide the definition of clinical supervision that will be used. This is a key step, as the definition should encapsulate the aims and approach that will be used and therefore provide an important step towards creating the shared vision that will be necessary for success. Agreeing to and disseminating a local definition is vital (McCallion and Baxter, 1995).

▶ The steps that have been taken so far should be developed by clearly describing the model of clinical supervision that is to be used. This may be done through taking an 'off the peg' approach by selecting one of the models described elsewhere in this book (see Chapter 3), adapting an existing model to suit local circumstances (Wright et al, 1997), or creating your own model based on your particular needs. The second of these three options is probably the most appropriate for the majority of circumstances. In order to maintain the involvement of the rest of the team (those who will use the model of clinical supervision) it would be useful at this point to explain how the selected model or approach will meet the objectives of the first stage.

▶ Once the project group is clear about its intentions there will be a need to identify resource and educational requirements. The educational/training needs will need to be carefully thought through. As discussed earlier, one of the concerns of those who will be expected to be supervising others will be in relation to their perceptions of the skills needed to fulfil this role. No assumptions can be made about the abilities of potential supervisors and such concerns must not be underestimated. Furthermore, those who are potential supervisees will also need to participate in the training; one needs preparation to get the most out of clinical supervision (Jones, 1998). Resourcing will be a major barrier to implementation if it is not adequately addressed. It will be difficult to calculate an exact financial cost at this stage. One illustration of the potential costs incurred comes from a director of nursing who estimated that the annual costs of implementing a monthly two-hour period of clinical supervision for every nurse in her district general hospital would be in the region of £100,000 (Smith, 1995). In order to establish resource and training requirements the minimum amount of supervision time for each nurse will need to be established and the criteria for designated supervisors defined.

From these initial stages you should emerge with some broad ideas that will most logically fall under three headings (Jones, 1998):

▶ Supervisor issues and needs.

▶ Supervisee issues and needs.

▶ Organisational issues (such as impact on workload, shift arrangements and so on).

If the principle of participation and involvement is to be maintained, it would be appropriate at this stage to open up the discussion through either open meetings or focus groups where the broad aims of clinical supervision, as defined by the team, and the strategy can be put forward.

These meetings can be supported, for example by ward or department-based newsletters and, if deemed appropriate, throughout the rest of the trust by poster displays and articles in trust-wide newsletters. As success is going to be dependent on team support it will be important to ensure a high profile is maintained until it becomes established.

The key purpose of such meetings will be to ensure that concerns are addressed and not allowed to become established barriers. (One approach to take with this is given in Case Study 1.)

The main concerns to be aware of and to take steps to manage will be as follows:

The concern that this is being driven through from above

While the decision to implement clinical supervision may be taken by the trust board/director of nursing as a consequence of the impetus from the NHSE, the UKCC's recommendation is that each clinical area should develop a tailor-made model that is appropriate to its needs (UKCC, 1996). Nevertheless, most staff will not see it as a 'grass roots' initiative. The way to overcome these concerns is to be open about them, recognise and acknowledge them, and to involve all staff at the earliest opportunity. The trust may have already sought to achieve this sense of ownership and participation by giving departments or clinical areas complete freedom to choose a model that meets their needs (with some provisos), or by adopting a model for the whole of the organisation that could easily be customised by the various clinical teams.

Even where there is a high degree of decision-making by clinical teams over the type of clinical supervision being introduced, there will be some decisions that will need to be taken either at directorate or trust management level. These will concern the resource implications of the proposed model since costs will be generated both by the need to adequately train supervisors and through the requirement of time for supervisor meetings. At present it is difficult to predict how much time will be needed for supervision (Porter, 1998).

The concerns of those who are going to be supervisors

For clinical supervision to be successful those who are to be supervisors will need preparation in the form of education and training.

It has been argued that the skills required to be a successful supervisor can be centred on restorative, formative and normative functions (Butterworth, 1994). Such skills will need to be developed and staff will have genuine concerns about what will be expected of them. Supervisors will also be concerned about accountability and confidentiality. 'What if I had supervised Beverly Allitt?' (Clothier et al, 1994) may well be an unspoken concern for many as the responsibilities associated with clinical supervision become apparent. Those who are to be supervisors will need to feel they have support; during the initial stages this support will focus more on the development of skills required to provide supervision. This type of support will need to be visible and should include the opportunity to attend formal taught programmes (Wright et al, 1997; Rafferty and Coleman, 1996).

Support for supervisors will also need to be provided on an ongoing basis and all supervisors themselves should be provided with supervision (Wright et al, 1997). This will ensure that there is an opportunity for the supervisors to develop their skills and discuss any issues raised by supervisees that they might wish to explore further.

The concerns of those who will be supervisees

As previously suggested, supervisees are likely to have concerns related to the extent to which this will be used as a form of managerial control, but they may also have concerns about confidentiality. As discussed, clinical supervision will not be successful unless those participating have the confidence to be open and honest. The message that must be got across when the selected model of clinical supervision is being introduced is that 'this is your tool; this is to help you to maintain and develop the things that will help you in your work'.

The concerns that staff might have about clinical supervision being a 'management tool' could be resolved by making supervision an advisory rather than a compulsory activity. This would have a number of benefits. It would allow the whole programme to be introduced at a pace that would match the development of supervisors, thereby avoiding a 'mad rush' for supervision early on. It would also result in members of the team who felt positive about the initiative receiving supervision first. These individuals would be more likely to feel that clinical supervision was of benefit to them, and they would be more likely to generate a positive view of supervision within the team.

The supervisee may also have concerns about who will be their supervisor. Just as imposing clinical supervision on an individual may create resistance, so there may be situations where 'imposing' a particular supervisor is unhelpful. The approach to selecting supervisors for staff will therefore need some consideration, both in terms of the choice of grade and in terms of matching individual supervisors and supervisees (Webb, 1997). Decisions regarding the issue of choice of grade and any implied hierarchical considerations should ideally be made with the involvement of the whole team. For example, the need for supervisees not to perceive clinical supervision as having a controlling function may be addressed by providing individual supervision from within the same grade. However, the real issue is less about grade but rather the competency/ability of the individual to provide supervision. These criteria are likely to be based around the experience, knowledge, competence and confidence of the intended supervisor. It would be appropriate for the team to further define the qualities that are appropriate within their area of practice.

Other concerns could be managed by acknowledging that team members should have some say in their choice of supervisor, although there would be a need to reach some common position on this to ensure that the supervision exercise is not an informal chat with a friend in the workplace.

The concerns about documentation

Given the strong emphasis placed on thorough documentation in nursing, both supervisor and supervisee might have anxieties about the nature and quality of any documentation arising from supervision meetings. Staff should be assured that there is no need for this level of formal documentation; supervision is not appraisal. Discussion is more likely to be open and able to examine meaningful issues if there is confidence that it will not be shared elsewhere (Burrow, 1995). Nevertheless, there will be the need to audit the process since organisations are unlikely to invest in clinical supervision without being satisfied that it is improving the service. The auditing might be undertaken formally by the trust. Equally, there may be an opportunity for the team itself to develop its own audit tool, which might be able to demonstrate the benefits of clinical supervision to staff on the ward as well as trust board members (see Chapter 8). Burrow (1995) suggests that the audit will be required to, among other things, monitor effectiveness, appraise outcomes and justify supervisory time.

CASE STUDIES

The following case studies demonstrate how the principles outlined so far can be applied to the practice setting.

Case study 1: Fostering team ownership and identifying concerns

In response to the NHS Executive guidance on clinical governance, the Dobcroft NHS Trust decided to introduce clinical supervision for nurses in all its directorates. Each directorate was issued with an internal memorandum stating that it must introduce a form of clinical supervision that was relevant to the needs of the nursing staff within six months. No model of supervision was suggested but the memorandum contained the names of individuals who had agreed to act as a resource to the trust's nurse managers. These were nurses who had some experience with clinical supervision within the region.

When Sue Smyth, director of nursing for the (six-ward) medical directorate received the memorandum she had immediate concerns about the time scale. On speaking to other directors of nursing within the trust she found that others also had this concern. Most of them had identified H grades within their directorates and given them the responsibility of introducing a clinical supervision model.

Sue was keen to involve the directorate staff as much as possible in any change that was being introduced but had sometimes found it difficult to generate involvement in a workforce that was, she felt, becoming cynical about change. She feared that this might be the case with the introduction of clinical supervision.

Although Sue had her own ideas about clinical supervision she decided to contact one of the names on the list of 'regional experts'. She knew a couple of names on the list but decided to contact a number of individuals before making her decision. She did have some difficulties in contacting people but she found the fact that she ended up chatting on the phone to staff nurses about their views on clinical supervision useful. In the end she decided against inviting someone from another medical directorate because she felt that staff in her team might respond negatively to a suggestion that they should introduce clinical supervision in a particular way. Instead she opted for someone who worked in learning disabilities to speak to her staff.

Sue arranged two meetings for staff in her directorate – one for day staff and one for night staff. All ward staff were invited to attend, including clerical staff if they were interested. At each meeting she outlined the task the directorates had been set by the trust but stated clearly that she felt that clinical supervision would only work if all the staff were involved in its implementation. She introduced the outside speaker who gave a short but excellent talk on clinical supervision; she was enthusiastic but said that each team should adapt existing models of clinical supervision to develop their own.

Afterwards there was an opportunity for questions, but at this point Sue was worried that the thoughts and views of many of the staff at the meeting might be overlooked. She decided to pass round a pad of 'post it' stickers to all those at the meeting and asked them to write what they thought the three main problems with the introduction of clinical supervision might be. If staff could only think of one problem then they were asked to write that down. Sue was surprised at the enthusiasm the staff had for this exercise. She gathered in the responses and grouped them. The main problems were the time scale set by the trust, the staff's limited knowledge about clinical supervision and the time to do it. Next Sue decided to use a similar exercise to ask the staff how they felt these problems might be resolved. When she grouped the responses she found that staff felt that they should ask the trust for more time, that a working group should be established to develop a definition and model for the directorate, and that regular meetings should be arranged so that staff knew what was happening. This exercise was so successful that Sue decided to arrange other meetings and repeat it.

After the meetings Sue felt she had a much better understanding of the concerns of staff. She also felt that she had created a sense of shared ownership of the problem and that the team had collectively helped her understand how to develop a strategy for the introduction of clinical supervision. When she spoke to the trust's director of nursing she was able to demonstrate the success of her staff involvement exercise but also present a strong case for a longer time scale to introduce clinical supervision.

The time scale originally set by the trust was subsequently revised and this had a positive effect on the medical directorate staff who had seen that they could influence the change process. A project team was set up comprised of staff from the six medical wards. They carried out a similar exercise to that originally conducted by Sue to identify what the staff felt they wanted from clinical supervision. On the basis of these meetings and the responses from staff at the original meetings, a model of clinical supervision was developed and a strategy for introduction was formulated.

The approach to change that Sue had adopted generated such a high degree of enthusiasm among staff that when a decision had to be taken to pilot the model of clinical supervision for three months on one ward, the name of the ward had to be drawn out of a hat!

Examples of good practice evident in this scenario include the following:

▶ Appropriate use of recognised expertise.

▶ Creating a structure for engaging the team in the problem solving process.

▶ Developing good understanding of the concerns of the team in the lead person.

▶ Renegotiating time scales.

▶ Building on success and enthusiasm within the team.

Case study 2: Developing existing practice and dealing with concerns

A community-based trust decided to formalise its approach to clinical supervision. Clinical supervision was being practised informally within three teams with varying degrees of success. Rachel Graham, the primary care development manager, was given the responsibility for standardising the approach to clinical supervision and addressing some of the concerns that had been raised by the staff involved regarding documentation and supervisor development.

Rachel's first step was to assess the nature of the problem and to gauge staff experience of clinical supervision. She produced a questionnaire for all staff within the trust's integrated nursing/health visitor teams. Staff were asked: whether they had experienced clinical supervision; what it entailed in their experience (their definition); whether they had received or felt they needed any formal training either as a supervisor or supervisee; and what documentation they were using.

The audit yielded useful information. Many staff had limited experience of clinical supervision, although many stated that they had discussed it in the workplace. Where supervision was being used, the responses were positive in that staff felt that it was benefiting care delivery. Two members of staff were undertaking graduate programmes and had received some theoretical input regarding clinical supervision. However, the majority of staff said that they had limited understanding of clinical supervision and were keen to develop their knowledge by receiving more formal teaching. The questionnaire responses revealed that, with the odd exception, documentation was not being used. It was clear from the responses that some people were anxious about the fact that staff were not documenting their supervision meetings.

Rachel felt that the audit of current practice and attitudes was positive. Clinical supervision was seen in a positive light but staff wanted to have more formalised training, and the issue of documentation needed to be addressed so that staff could be reassured. A report of the assessment exercise was produced which reflected the findings and identified the concerns of staff. Rachel was also able to present the staff view of clinical supervision in a positive light. A supplementary question was attached to the report asking the teams who were not presently using supervision about their preferred time scale for its introduction.

Although the intention had been to standardise clinical supervision within the trust, it was apparent from the audit that it was being practised well within some teams. It was recognised that imposing a model on these teams would be counter-productive. What was needed was some clarification regarding supervisor practice and documentation, thereby addressing some of the anxieties and concerns.

Rachel arranged a meeting with the three teams that were currently practising clinical supervision and an invitation was extended to other interested parties within the trust. Each team briefly described its current practice and was asked to identify the areas that they felt needed development. (These were compatible with some of the responses from the original audit, but other issues were raised. It was evident that staff felt they should be able to discuss their concerns more openly.) The areas that staff felt required clarification were: training, frequency of meetings, whether they needed a theoretical model and issues concerning confidentiality and documentation.

These four issues were discussed within small groups following the initial discussion and identification of problems. The following solutions were proposed:

▶ Both supervisor and supervisee would receive training to develop their existing supervision arrangements.

▶ Supervision meetings should occur on a six-weekly basis and time should be set aside during the working day.

▶ A model of reflective practice was chosen. One of the staff had undertaken an assignment on Johns' reflective model (Johns, 1995) and agreed to present this to the group at the next meeting.

▶ All supervision meetings between supervisor and supervisee were to be confidential. Issues relating to possible unsafe practice would be resolved in accordance with a contract agreed by supervisor and supervisee.

Any documented notes from the meeting would be kept by the supervisee. There was some discussion regarding reflective diaries but the group agreed to return to this issue at a subsequent meeting. Documentation would be used to record whether supervision meetings took place and, if not, what the problem was. This would enable an audit of existing arrangements.

Rachel had been keen not to undermine what was already being practised and decided not to introduce the idea of a standardised approach by identifying one model of practice that was being used. It was clear that, through its own discussions, the working group was creating a mutual convergence of ideas. The broad principles were subsequently developed into a set of guidelines that could be used throughout the trust as each team introduced its own clinical supervision arrangements in accordance with the agreed time scale.

Examples of good practice evident in this scenario include the following:

▶ Assessing and auditing the problem.

▶ Building on the positive.

▶ Sharing experiences and ideas.

▶ Collaborative approach to resolving identified problems.

SUMMARY

As discussed in Chapter 5, the implementation of any change will have costs and benefits. The costs of introducing an organisational innovation such as clinical supervision into a busy working environment are most obviously seen in the time, energy and resources that are needed, but which may not be available. One of the advantages of the participative approach suggested here, is that it is more likely to generate the support needed to ensure successful implementation of the initiative. Staff will be more willing to engage in something of which they feel ownership.

The implementation strategy needs to be logically thought through but at the same time be flexible enough to respond to the needs and concerns of those most affected. This strategy should establish common ownership of the aims and purpose of clinical supervision for the area/directorate and ensure that everyone involved has a good understanding of the intentions.

It will be important to ensure that those leading the strategy have the necessary skills and knowledge to carry this through and to be prepared to seek appropriate support and guidance where required.

Recognising and acknowledging the concerns of the team members is essential whether they are supervisors or supervisees, particularly over the skills required to supervise, about confidentiality and about dealing with examples of poor practice.

The approach taken to documentation is likely to be crucial given these concerns, especially with regard to how it will be used to evaluate practice. However, for auditing purposes there will need to be some form of documentation, for example records of when supervision meetings take place or when they are cancelled. Personal documentation and records will most likely be at the discretion of both parties involved in the supervision process but should be encouraged as a tool for personal reflection and development.

Once a form of clinical supervision is agreed, both supervisor and supervisee will require preparation and training. Designated training days will make it possible to provide an overview for individuals, but their uptake may be limited given the demands of the service. A cascade approach to preparation may well offer advantages of flexibility, but to work effectively requires staff commitment.

Finally, the success or failure of clinical supervision will depend on a good level of trust and confidence in the process and on the enthusiasm and support of all involved. This cannot be taken for granted but must be fostered by a well-planned and participative implementation process.

REFERENCES

Burrow, S. (1995) Supervision: clinical development or management control. *British Journal of Nursing*; 4: 15, 879–882.

Butterworth, T. (1994) Preparing to take on clinical supervision. *Nursing Standard*; 21: 8, 32–34.

Clothier, C., MacDonald, C.A., Shaw, D.A. (1994) *The Allitt Enquiry*. London: HMSO.

Coch, L., French, J.R.P. (1948) Overcoming resistance to change. *Human Relations*; 1, 512–532.

Dunphy, D.C., Stace, D.A. (1990) *Under New Management: Australian Organisations in Transition*. Sydney: McGraw-Hill.

Goorapah, D. (1997) Clinical supervision. *Journal of Clinical Nursing*; 6: 3, 173–178.

Johns, C. (1995) Value of reflective practice for nursing. *Journal of Clinical Nursing*; 4, 23–30.

Jones, A. (1998) Getting going with clinical supervision: an introductory seminar. *Journal of Advanced Nursing*; 27: 3, 560–566.

Likert, R. (1961) *New Patterns of Management*. New York, NY: McGraw-Hill.

McCallion, H., Baxter, T. (1995) Clinical supervision: take it from the top. *Nursing Management*; 1: 10, 9.

McGregor, D. (1987) *The Human Side of Enterprise*. London: Penguin.

Pasmore, W., Friedlander, F. (1982) An action research programme to increase employee involvement 1: problem solving. *Administrative Science Quarterly*; 27: 3, 343–362.

Porter, N. (1998) Providing effective clinical supervision. *Nursing Management*; 5: 2, 22–23.

Rafferty, M., Coleman, M. (1996) Educating nurses to undertake clinical supervision in practice. *Nursing Standard*; 10: 45, 38–41.

Smith, J. (1995) Clinical supervision: conference organised by NHS Executive (Conference Report). *Journal of Advanced Nursing*; 21: 5, 1029–1031.

United Kingdom Central Council for Nursing, Midwifery and Health Visiting (1996) *Position Statement on Clinical Supervision for Nursing and Health Visiting*. London: UKCC.

Webb, B. (1997) Auditing a clinical supervision training programme. *Nursing Standard*; 11: 34, 34–39.

Wright, S., Elliot, M., Schofield, H. (1997) A networking approach to clinical supervision. *Nursing Standard*; 11: 18, 39–41.

8 Making clinical supervision happen

Chris Bassett

It is clear that clinical supervision is important in helping staff learn and develop their care and as a method to help reduce stress. It is hoped that after reading and reflecting on this guide you will feel able to begin implementation of clinical supervision in your area of practice. Throughout the book the authors have given advice and hints on achieving success. It is, of course, important to follow the principles for effective change when implementing any new innovation or practice, and clinical supervision is no different.

STEPS FOR SUCCESS

- ▶ A clear and open approach to implementation is essential.
- ▶ The benefits of supervision must be made clear to all members of the team.
- ▶ For clinical supervision to work properly it must be embraced by all members of the team.

A crucial part of the implementation of clinical supervision is the preparation phase and the provision of training prior to supervision being fully introduced. It is the preparation for training and a practical exploration of the key issues that I will now briefly describe, as well as offering some suggestions on how clinical supervision training might be carried out successfully. There are several key issues to take into consideration.

When implementing clinical supervision in any area it is important to identify the basic principles relating to its use and success in the clinical setting.

- ▶ Supervision should become part and parcel of professional nursing or healthcare practice.
- ▶ It should begin with basic professional education and continue as an integral part of professional development.
- ▶ It requires time, commitment and energy.
- ▶ Organisational commitment is implicit.
- ▶ Supervision should be protected in times of financial difficulty.
- ▶ Clinical supervision does not have one model and must be flexible to reflect specific areas.
- ▶ Practitioners must develop their own ways of supervising each other.
- ▶ Clinical supervision must be locally led.

All of the above factors must be supported by nurse managers if clinical supervision is to have any chance of success (Farrington, 1996). Another important point to bear in mind is the fact that clinical supervision is closely linked with reflective practice; both go hand in hand with improving morale and creating a learning organisation (Fox, 1994). To support supervision it is important to consider reflective practice and to understand the key issues.

EDUCATION AND TRAINING FOR CLINICAL SUPERVISION

As with any new innovation a comprehensive training and education period is essential for a successful outcome (Nightingale, 1997). The first issues to address are who needs to be trained and how long the training should last. My personal view is that everyone who is to participate in clinical supervision must be included in the training – both trained and untrained. It is important to be aware of the benefits and responsibilities that come with supervision. It must be remembered that each member of the team will be both a supervisor and a supervisee. Each of these roles will have a slightly different emphasis attached to it. Therefore, it is important that these roles are clearly defined within the training programme (Cerinus and Ferguson, 1994). The next issue that must be decided is the length of training required. There are obvious difficulties when considering time for training. There are many different needs competing for limited time: PREP needs, individual performance reviews, team and unit meetings. How long is best? Some trainers would advocate three to five days as a minimum for training; others would say half a day is sufficient. My own view is that one day is possibly a good compromise and one that can be achieved (Bassett, 1999).

What follows now are suggestions that could be included as part of a training day designed to help prepare nurses for clinical supervision.

Clinical supervision training

Introduction to the subject of clinical supervision

This will include the key documents outlining the need for a formalised approach to supervision.

Group work: exploring the benefits of clinical supervision

Break the group up into smaller units to consider the following:

What are the benefits for the

▶ patient

▶ staff member

▶ organisation

with clinical supervision running effectively in the trust?

Group work: exploring the key issues and potential problems relating to clinical supervision

Issues raised may include:

▶ Who supervises whom?

▶ Problems with relationships.

▶ Time constraints.

▶ Ethical dilemmas.

▶ Where supervision may take place.

At all stages it is important to encourage course members to brainstorm issues and problems and help them find possible solutions to problems.

Following the identification of perceived problems it is important to spend time exploring the issues raised. This will help the course members to think about ways that they can help supervision take place.

Formal session on choosing a supervisor

The next area to consider might be how a supervisor will be chosen. Will it be a superior or a peer that is the best person to supervise? Does the supervisor need to be from the same profession? What about team leaders and ward sisters – who will supervise them?

It is very important to focus on the problems as time spent here may save time later.

Ethical issues and confidentiality

Again it will be important to consider 'what ifs'. For instance, 'What if a supervisor breaks confidentiality?' The key to supervision is clearly that staff must trust each other. Supervision will only be of value if participants can be sure that what they say is secret. Once confidentiality is broken, the trust that is essential to support clinical supervision is lost. However, there are also issues such as, 'What if a supervisee discloses something that may be unsafe or dangerous practice, or indeed criminal?' This is clearly different and the UKCC code of conduct really points the way forward here. This leads neatly into the next important issue, that is the setting of clear and effective guidelines prior to the supervision process taking place.

Setting ground rules

One of the most effective ways of ensuring a level of success is the negotiation between parties of clear and succinct ground rules. These rules will include the following issues:

- How frequent will the meetings be?
- What will the limits of discussion be?
- How long will the meetings last?
- What happens if one of us keeps missing the session?

By pre-empting these potential problems the chance of failure will be reduced.

Finally, it may be useful to break the group up into pairs to begin to consider the creation of ground rules with each other. The pairs can then explore the issues surrounding the practicalities of ensuring sustained and effective clinical supervision.

GAINING SUPPORT FOR CHANGE

There can be little doubt that for the nurse implementing clinical supervision this can be a very difficult process. It is also true, however, that in order for nursing care to move on clinical supervision must become part of our working lives. This section aims to provide you with insights and practical advice on how support for change can be identified and built on.

Making clinical supervision stick

Change is about selling. It is about how enthusiastic people, who have a powerful idea or vision of how things could be better organised or done, get sometimes less enthusiastic people to try to implement their idea. When translated into nursing it is usually about a nurse, or group of nurses, who wants to introduce a new type of nursing practice or innovation. As mentioned above, this can be a very hard thing to do. My personal experience of change is that it can be at times demoralising, at times frustrating, at times energy sapping, but never dull. And sometimes, when a change has been adopted and proven of value it is really rewarding. This is the case with clinical supervision.

Keeping going

I am sure that you will be fully aware of the difficulties with starting and maintaining change. If you are not absolutely determined to overcome all possible barriers in your way, then stop reading right now. If you believe that in order for nurses to give the very best care to their patients you must make changes, then read on as we consider the ways that support for clinical supervision can be found and utilised.

Constraints to change

As mentioned in the chapters on change, there are many specific factors involved in overcoming barriers to clinical supervision. These include:

▶ the size of the required change;

▶ level of ritualistic practice in the area;

▶ perceived cost of the change;

▶ obstructive colleagues – could be nurses or doctors;

▶ low morale;

▶ apathy;

▶ poor communication;

▶ poor leadership.

This list is not exhaustive and there may be many other factors involved. However, from this exercise it is easier to see the difficulties that you will need to overcome if you wish to make clinical supervision happen.

Supporting factors

As mentioned previously, change is notoriously hard to achieve but there are many ways available to support change. Obviously, success may depend on the level and diversity of support available. Examples of supporting factors are:

▶ supportive team;

▶ supportive managers;

▶ open and listening culture in the ward or department;

▶ good communication;

▶ high morale;

▶ accessible and interested link teacher or educationalists;

▶ knowledge of change theories;

▶ understanding of the research process.

There will doubtless be many other avenues of support to identify and pursue.

Supportive teamwork

Clearly, this is easier if you are part of a clinical supervision implementation team. If you are not, however, it is important to try to foster a team approach in the people you are aiming to help with the change. The way that you choose to make the change is, of course, important and will ultimately affect the ease or difficulty of the process.

Supportive managers

Your managers, whether they are first line or middle managers, have a great influence on the effectiveness of the implementation of clinical supervision. It is easy to knock management, but generally they are delighted to see that members of staff are motivated enough to innovate and explore new approaches that support their nursing care. They are driven by the same evidence-based imperatives as all healthcare professionals. They will more than likely see you as an ally helping to develop their area. The key issues are to involve the manager in the process, to let them know why you feel clinical supervision should be implemented and what benefits might be gained. They may be able to either free you up with more time or assist with some (usually small) funding or secretarial support.

An open and learning ward culture

Implementing clinical supervision is undoubtedly easier when the environment and culture of the ward or department is based on principles of openness. With the help of others, you need to develop a questioning approach to practice, and one that values the views of all members of the team.

Good communication

It follows that if you have good, clear paths of communication both up and down the ward structure, then you stand a much greater chance of stimulating clinical supervision. The message must be clear; ambiguity is likely to slow things down. Benefits to the patients and staff must be made clear as well as the ways that success might be measured. You and the staff cannot be sure that you have achieved success if a measure of that success has not been identified early on in the process.

High morale

If you have a high performing team then anything is possible. High morale is not a thing of the past that old-style nurses reminisce about; it still exists. It can be built on and enhanced by fostering a team spirit and by plenty of personal enthusiasm. With a robust system of clinical supervision you will find that all members of staff will work together and patient care will improve. You can help foster an environment that stimulates general change by a good clinical supervision programme.

Knowledge of change theories and the research process

These two concepts are closely related. It is perhaps obvious that a great support for the nurse involved in clinical supervision is a detailed and in-depth knowledge of the theories of change. There are many courses offered by universities or in-service training departments that provide a chance for further study of this important subject. Change has been identified as one of the key knowledge areas required by all nurses (Smith and Bassett, 1996). It is worthwhile considering again the great rewards that can be gained, not just from improved patient care and job satisfaction but through a really strong personal sense of achievement, when you have helped implement clinical supervision in your practice area. Change can be exceedingly hard to achieve but with a carefully structured, considered and enthusiastic approach you will definitely achieve it.

REFERENCES

Bassett, C. (1999) Clinical supervision in perioperative practice. *British Journal of Theatre Nursing*; 9: 7, 297–300.

Cerinus, M., Ferguson, C. (1994) Preparing nurses for preceptorship. *Nursing Standard*; 3: 16, 805.

Cutcliffe, J., Proctor, B. (1998) An alternative training approach to clinical supervision. *British Journal of Nursing*; 7: 5, 280–284.

Farrington, A. (1996) Clinical supervision. *British Journal of Nursing*; 5: 12, 716.

Fox, J. (1994) Clinical supervision: a real aspiration. *British Journal of Nursing*; 8: 36, 34–38.

Middleman, R., Rhodes, G. (1985) *Competent Supervision: Making Imaginative Judgements*. Englewood Cliffs, NJ: Prentice-Hall.

Nightingale, K. (1997) You, the clinical supervisor. *British Journal of Theatre Nursing*; 6: 10, 21.

Smith, L. Bassett, C. (1996) Introducing change into the post-anaesthetic care unit. *Nursing Standard*; 11: 9, 36–38.

Wilkin, P., Bowers, L., Monk, J. (1997) A network approach to clinical supervision. *Nursing Standard*; 11: 18, 39–41.

Index